T0362316

Quality in Thoracic Surgery

Editor

FELIX G. FERNANDEZ

THORACIC SURGERY CLINICS

www.thoracic.theclinics.com

Consulting Editor
M. BLAIR MARSHALL

August 2017 • Volume 27 • Number 3

ELSEVIER

1600 John F. Kennedy Boulevard ● Suite 1800 ● Philadelphia, Pennsylvania, 19103-2899

http://www.thoracic.theclinics.com

THORACIC SURGERY CLINICS Volume 27, Number 3
August 2017 ISSN 1547-4127, ISBN-13; 978-0-323-53259-4

Editor: John Vassallo (j.vassallo@elsevier.com)
Developmental Editor: Colleen Dietzler

Thoracic Surgery Clinics (ISSN 1547-4127) is published quarterly by Elsevier Inc., 360 Park Avenue South, New York, NY 10010-1710. Months of publication are February, May, August, and November. Business and editorial offices: 1600 John F. Kennedy Boulevard, Suite 1800, Philadelphia, PA 19103-2899. Periodicals postage paid at New York, NY, and additional mailing offices. Subscription prices are $359.00 per year (US individuals), $521.00 per year (US institutions), $100.00 per year (US Students), $439.00 per year (Canadian individuals), $674.00 per year (Canadian institutions), $225.00 per year (Canadian and international students), $470.00 per year (international individuals), and $674.00 per year (international institutions). Foreign air speed delivery is included in all Clinics' subscription prices. All prices are subject to change without notice. **POSTMASTER:** Send address changes to Thoracic Surgery Clinics, Elsevier Health Sciences Division, Subscription Customer Service, 3251 Riverport Lane, Maryland Heights, MO 63043. **Customer Service (orders, claims, online, change of address): Telephone: 1-800-654-2452 (U.S. and Canada); 314-447-8871 (outside U.S. and Canada). Fax: 314-447-8029. E-mail: journalscustomerservice-usa@elsevier.com (for print support); journalsonlinesupport-usa@elsevier.com (for online support).**

Reprints. For copies of 100 or more, of articles in this publication, please contact Commercial Rights Department, Elsevier Inc., 360 Park Avenue South, New York, NY 10010-1710. Tel: 212-633-3874; Fax: 212-633-3820; E-mail: reprints@elsevier.com.

Thoracic Surgery Clinics is covered in *MEDLINE/PubMed (Index Medicus), EMBASE/Excerpta Medica, Science Citation Index Expanded (SciSearch®), Journal Citation Reports/Science Edition,* and *Current Contents®/Clinical Medicine.*

Contributors

CONSULTING EDITOR

M. BLAIR MARSHALL, MD, FACS
Chief, Division of Thoracic Surgery, Associate
Professor, Department of Surgery,
Georgetown University Medical Center,
Georgetown University School of Medicine,
Washington, DC

EDITOR

FELIX G. FERNANDEZ, MD, MSc
Associate Professor of Surgery, Section of
General Thoracic Surgery, Emory University
School of Medicine, The Emory Clinic, Atlanta,
Georgia

AUTHORS

ALESSANDRO BRUNELLI, MD
Department of Thoracic Surgery, St. James's
University Hospital, Leeds, United Kingdom

WILLIAM R. BURFEIND Jr, MD
Clinical Associate Professor of
Surgery, Temple University School of
Medicine, Department of Surgery, St. Luke's
University Health Network, Bethlehem,
Pennsylvania

ANDREW C. CHANG, MD
Head, Section of Thoracic Surgery,
Department of Surgery, University of Michigan,
Ann Arbor, Michigan

ANTHONY CIPRIANO, MD
Department of Surgery, St. Luke's
University Health Network, Bethlehem,
Pennsylvania

PIERRE-EMMANUEL FALCOZ, MD, PhD
Department of Thoracic Surgery, Nouvel
Hospital Civil, University of Strasborg,
Strasbourg, France

FARHOOD FARJAH, MD, MPH
Associate Professor of Surgery, Division of
Cardiothoracic Surgery, University of
Washington, Seattle, Washington

FELIX G. FERNANDEZ, MD, MSc
Associate Professor of Surgery, Section of
General Thoracic Surgery, Emory University
School of Medicine, The Emory Clinic, Atlanta,
Georgia

SETH D. FORCE, MD
Professor of Surgery, Chief, General Thoracic
Surgery, Section of General Thoracic Surgery,
Division of Cardiothoracic Surgery, Emory
University School of Medicine, Atlanta, Georgia

RICHARD K. FREEMAN, MD, MBA
Department of Thoracic and Cardiovascular
Surgery, St Vincent Hospital, Indianapolis,
Indiana

JESSICA HUDSON, MD, MSc
Resident Physician, Department of
Cardiothoracic Surgery, Washington University
School of Medicine, St Louis, Missouri

ONKAR V. KHULLAR, MD
Assistant Professor of Surgery,
Section of General Thoracic Surgery,
Emory University School of Medicine, Atlanta,
Georgia

BENJAMIN D. KOZOWER, MD, MPH
Professor of Surgery, Washington University
School of Medicine, St Louis, Missouri

MITCHELL J. MAGEE, MD, MSc
Chief, Division of Thoracic Surgery, Medical
City Dallas Hospital, Dallas, Texas

RACHEL L. MEDBERY, MD
Thoracic Surgery Fellow, Section of General
Thoracic Surgery, Division of Cardiothoracic
Surgery, Emory University School of Medicine,
Atlanta, Georgia

VARUN PURI, MD, MSCI
Associate Professor, Department of
Cardiothoracic Surgery, Washington University
School of Medicine, St Louis, Missouri

DANIEL P. RAYMOND, MD, FACS, FCCP
Chief Quality Officer, Thoracic Surgery,
Cleveland Clinic Foundation, Cleveland, Ohio

MICHELE SALATI, MD
Ospedali Riuniti Ancona, Ancona, Italy

CHRISTOPHER W. SEDER, MD
Department of Cardiovascular and Thoracic
Surgery, Rush University Medical Center,
Chicago, Illinois

TARA SEMENKOVICH, MD
Resident Physician, Department of
Cardiothoracic Surgery, Washington University
School of Medicine, St Louis, Missouri

GEORGE J. STUKENBORG, PhD
Professor of Public Health Sciences, University
of Virginia School of Medicine, Charlottesville,
Virginia

STEPHANIE G. WORRELL, MD
Cardiothoracic Surgery Fellow, Section of
Thoracic Surgery, University of Michigan,
Ann Arbor, Michigan

Contents

Comparative audit is an essential tool for multicenter quality efforts. The components include a rigorously defined and collected data source, carefully selected and defined preintervention patient variables that may impact outcome, appropriate risk stratification to aid in comparing varying populations, meticulous outcome selection and analysis, and independent audit to ensure the veracity of the data.

Achieving high-quality care for all patients undergoing esophageal cancer requires identifying and modifying risk factors associated with poor outcomes. These factors occur at different time points from the preoperative to the postoperative periods. A straightforward model for predicting outcomes has proved difficult to identify. This article reviews the current studies addressing risk adjustment and performance measurement for esophageal cancer resection.

This article outlines a structure for assessing thoracic surgical quality and provides an overview of evidence-based quality metrics for surgical care in both lung cancer and esophageal cancer, with a focus on process and outcome measures in the preoperative, intraoperative, and postoperative setting.

The National Quality Forum (NQF) is a multistakeholder, nonprofit, membership-based organization improving health care through preferential use of valid performance measures. NQF-endorsed measures are considered the gold standard for health care measurement in the United States. The Society of Thoracic Surgeons is the steward of the only six NQF-endorsed general thoracic surgery measures. These measures include one structure measure (participation in a national general thoracic surgery database), two process measures (recording of clinical stage and recording performance status before lung and esophageal resections), and three outcome measures (risk-adjusted morbidity and mortality after lung and esophageal resections and risk-adjusted length of stay greater than 14 days after lobectomy).

Most thoracic surgery studies indicate that hospital and surgeon procedure volume are inversely associated with mortality. However, controversy exists regarding the strength and validity of this volume-outcome association. Because thresholds of procedure volume are used to recommend the regionalization of care, investigation of the volume-outcome relationship is imperative. This article examines the methodology used in the volume-outcome relationship literature and highlights important areas of concern. Careful examination of the literature demonstrates that lung and esophageal cancer resection volume is not strongly associated with mortality and should not be used as a proxy measure for quality.

Variability in outcomes not attributable to case mix or chance is an indicator of low-quality care. Failure-to-rescue is an outcome measure defined as death during a hospitalization among patients who experience a complication. Researchers have used this measure to better understand the determinants of an untimely death—preventing complications, rescue, or both. Studies repeatedly find that complication rates vary little, if at all, across hospitals ranked by risk-adjusted mortality rates, suggesting that hospitals are equally capable (or incapable) of preventing complications. In contrast, variation in failure-to-rescue rates seems to explain much of the variation in risk-adjusted hospital-level mortality rates. These findings suggest that system-level interventions that allow for the early detection and treatment of complications (ie, rescue) may reduce variability in hospital-level outcomes and improve the quality of thoracic surgical care.

The value of health care is defined as health outcomes (quality) achieved per dollars spent (cost). The current national health care landscape is focused on minimizing spending while optimizing patient outcomes. With the introduction of minimally invasive thoracic surgery, there has been concern about added cost relative to improved outcomes. Moreover, differences in postoperative hospital care further drive patient outcomes and health care costs. This article presents a comprehensive literature review on quality and cost in thoracic surgery and aims to investigate current challenges with regard to achieving the greatest value for our patients.

The existing thoracic surgical literature contains several retrospective and observational studies that include patient-reported outcomes. To deliver true patient-centered care, it will be necessary to universally gather patient-reported outcomes prospectively, including them in routine patient care, clinical registries, and clinical trials.

Administrative data are less accurate and relevant than specialty-specific, procedure-specific, risk-adjusted data collected in voluntary registries such as the Society of Thoracic Surgeons-General Thoracic Surgery Database (GTSD). Voluntary clinical databases must be proven accurate and complete before they are accepted as credible information sources. With substantial growth of the GTSD, an annual audit was initiated in 2010 to assess the completeness, accuracy, and quality of the data collected. The audit process is essential in validating data quality and adding credibility and value to volunteer clinical registries. It serves as an important tool for improvement of patient care.

THORACIC SURGERY CLINICS

RELATED INTEREST

Thoracic Surgery Clinics, November 2015 (Vol. 25, Issue 4)
Prevention and Management of Postoperative Complications
John D. Mitchell, *Editor*
Available at: http://www.thoracic.theclinics.com/

THE CLINICS ARE AVAILABLE ONLINE!
Access your subscription at:
www.theclinics.com

Preface
Quality in Thoracic Surgery

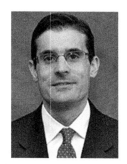

Felix G. Fernandez, MD, MSc
Editor

The field of quality measurement and quality improvement in health care continues to evolve. Multiple stakeholders, including patients, physicians, and payers, bring different perspectives as to what constitutes high-quality care. Assessments of quality are used to improve processes of care, rank providers, guide patient choice, and guide reimbursement. Historically, quality in surgical care has been measured with the hard clinical endpoints of morbidity and mortality. While such outcome measures are still valid, other measures, such as patient quality of life, cost, and resource utilization, are critical and must be measured. At present, our ability to collect, analyze, and use these data is a matter that is meaningful to our patients, and health systems remain limited. In this issue of *Thoracic Surgery Clinics*, an expert group of thoracic surgeons with a specific interest in quality measurement and improvement provides a detailed review of the current state and future directions of quality measurement in thoracic surgery.

Articles in this issue by Dr Raymond and Dr Chang and colleague, respectively, give an overview on current methodologies for risk assessment and performance measurement in lung and esophageal cancer surgery. Both of these experts have extensive experience in the development of such methodologies through the Society of Thoracic Surgeons (STS) General Thoracic Surgery Database (GTSD). Next, Dr Puri and colleagues explore the relevance of oncologic quality indicators in thoracic surgery, such as completeness of resection and lymph node staging. Such critical process measures are currently not included in many measures of performance

for lung and esophageal cancer surgery. National Quality Forum (NQF) –endorsed quality metrics in thoracic surgery are then reviewed in the article by Dr Burfeind, who has helped lead STS in the development of NQF quality metrics, and colleague.

The next four articles in this issue provide an overview of other surrogates or alternate measures of quality in surgery. Volume of surgical procedures performed has long been postulated as a marker of higher-quality care. Dr Kozower, who has significant experience investigating this topic, provides an in-depth analysis of the relevance of volume outcome relationships in thoracic surgery. Dr Farjah explores the "failure to rescue" outcome metric to distinguish high- and low-quality thoracic surgery programs. Value in health care is often defined as quality divided by cost. Providers and health care entities seek to provide high quality while containing costs. In the article by Dr Force and colleague, the association with high-quality care in thoracic surgery and associated health care costs is described. Importantly, missing from our assessments of quality in surgery is the patient perspective. Dr Khullar and I provide an introduction to patient-reported outcomes and their relevance to quality measurement in thoracic surgery in our article.

The final articles of this issue cover several important topics. The veracity of our databases, in particular the STS GTSD, allows us to develop accurate risk models and performance measures. Dr Magee, who has led the audit of the GTSD for the STS, reports on the importance and results of the database audit process. Dr Brunelli next introduces the European Society of

Thorac Surg Clin 27 (2017) ix–x
http://dx.doi.org/10.1016/j.thorsurg.2017.05.001
1547-4127/17/© 2017 Published by Elsevier Inc.

Thoracic Surgeons (ESTS) database and risk models for thoracic surgery. In order to facilitate exchange of data and learning across societies, the STS and ESTS have engaged in a database collaboration. Drs Seder and Salati describe the impetus and nature of this collaboration as well as the opportunities this will provide for advancement of the field of thoracic surgery. Finally, Dr Freeman discusses the often scrutinized metric of hospital readmissions following thoracic surgery.

Quality in thoracic surgery consists of many components: the safety of the surgery, long-term survival and quality of life, and containment of costs and resource utilization. An expert group of thoracic surgeons has contributed thoughtful scholarly reviews on various topics related to the field of quality measurement. I hope that you enjoy their contributions and enhance your understanding of quality measurement.

Felix G. Fernandez, MD, MSc
The Emory Clinic
1365 Clifton Road, Northeast, Suite A2214
Atlanta, GA 30322, USA

E-mail address:
felix.fernandez@emoryhealthcare.org

Risk Adjustment and Performance Measurement for Lung Cancer Resection

Daniel P. Raymond, MD

KEYWORDS

- Risk stratification • Outcome measurement • Quality • Lung surgery

KEY POINTS

- Risk stratification requires the collection of rigorously defined variables from a reliable data source.
- Variables should ideally be objective, reliably collected, inexpensive to acquire, and have appropriate variation in the patient population being examined.
- The complexity and cost of each variable needs to be carefully considered before inclusion in any multiinstitutional quality effort.

INTRODUCTION

Comparative audit is an essential tool for multi-center quality efforts. The components include a rigorously defined and collected data source, carefully selected and defined preintervention patient variables that may impact outcome, appropriate risk stratification to aid in comparing varying populations, meticulous outcome selection and analysis, and independent audit to ensure the veracity of the data.

RISK STRATIFICATION

Risk stratification is an essential tool for clinical decision making as well as a standardization tool for comparative audit. The latter is an essential feature of performance enhancement because benchmarks are vital to the development of quality improvement efforts. Essential to risk assessment for comparative audit is first clearly defining an outcome measure. This metric ideally is a clearly defined, objective measure that is relatively simple to collect. This outcome must occur with a reasonable frequency in the population being examined to provide a meaningful analysis that differentiates the performance of contributing entities. Once an outcome is chosen, the risk assessment begins generally with a determination of variables, based on expert consensus and past clinical data that may have a causative relationship with the outcome in question. Inherently, risk stratification models are best suited for the initial purpose designed. Extrapolation outside the original design must be validated to ensure accuracy. For instance, the Charlson Comorbidity Index[1] was developed to predict 10-year mortality in medical patients. The application to other patient populations has resulted in variable efficacy, which often leads to modifications such as reweighting of the variables.[2,3] Furthermore, risk models are susceptible to "calibration drift."[4] Simply put, this is the potential impact of therapeutic evolution on risk modeling over time. A good example would be the revolutionary development of antiviral medication for the treatment of hepatitis C and the impact on risk models for liver failure.

Ideal variables chosen for risk assessment have several common characteristics listed in **Box 1**. There are basically three types of risk

The author has no financial disclosures relevant to this article.
Thoracic Surgery, Cleveland Clinic Foundation, 9500 Euclid Avenue, J4-1, Cleveland, OH 44195, USA
E-mail address: raymond3@ccf.org

Thorac Surg Clin 27 (2017) 215–220
http://dx.doi.org/10.1016/j.thorsurg.2017.03.001

Box 1
Ideal characteristics of variables chosen for risk assessment or outcome measurement

1. Objective
2. Reliably collected
3. Inexpensive to acquire
4. Not complex
5. Appropriate variation in the population being evaluated

factors: (1) objective, (2) subjective, and (3) patient reported. Clearly, objective measures have the greatest value because they are least susceptible to bias. There is value, however, in subjective and patient-reported variables. An interesting example of the value of subjectivity is the American Society of Anesthesia Physical Status classification. The Society of Anesthesia Physical Status classification is a simple severity of illness scoring system that generally provides good discrimination for predicting postoperative mortality in a broad range of patients.[4] This finding is likely owing to the subjective nature of the scoring system, which permits the practitioner to collate numerous clinical variables including functional status in a single score. Admittedly, however, the score has been shown only to have moderate interrater reliability.[5]

Furthermore, variables for risk assessment should be reliably and inexpensively collected. Variables that require extensive chart review or complex interpretation are not practical for large-scale data collection efforts. Certainly, technology can be an excellent means of automating and simplifying this process. For example, complex tests such as cardiopulmonary exercising testing may be an accurate means of assessing exercise tolerance before lung resection, but the cost and complexity of the examination does not justify application broadly at present. Furthermore, tests that require expertise to evaluate, such as reading radiologic studies, may not be practical owing to interobserver variation and the skill set required to critically review and record results. To ensure the accuracy of such tests, an audit system should be established by independent reviewers to ensure the accuracy of the reported variables.

Finally, variables chosen for risk assessment must occur with a reasonable frequency in the patient population being studied. Rare diagnoses that have significant impact on outcome create a challenge for any group attempting to risk stratify a population. A solution is to attempt to group these diagnoses among broader definitions, such as specific organ system dysfunction; however, this classification results in more ambiguity of the definition and requires more complex data interpretation by data collectors. One could argue that these types of diagnoses should occur with a relatively similar frequency as a whole in the patient population and thus balance out the risk. In contrast, the designation of centers as tertiary and quaternary with specific referral patterns argues against this assumption.

The Society of Thoracic Surgery (STS) has done an excellent job of risk stratifying patients undergoing lobectomy for lung cancer resection.[6,7] There are clearly defined outcome measures, including major morbidity, mortality and combined morbidity and mortality after lobectomy for lung cancer. The risk stratification includes a broad list of more than 30 variables with succinct definitions provided by the STS for accurate data acquisition. These data are used to construct a risk model that has identified significant predictors of postoperative outcomes. Furthermore, this model was used to provide a comparative audit of contributor's performance. The distribution of performances demonstrates statistical significance between the highest and lowest performers, suggesting the model provides useful discrimination.

Notably, this model has been updated to accommodate for the possibility of calibration drift.[7] Encouragingly, the first update of the model demonstrated a surprising decline in operative mortality (from 2.2% in 2002–2008 to 1.4% in 2012–2014),[6] suggesting the quality efforts by the STS have led to meaningful improvements in surgical outcomes for participants.

A critical review of this risk assessment does, however, identify opportunities for improvement. The preoperative variables include several common diagnosis such as diabetes mellitus, peripheral vascular disease, and congestive heart failure. This list, understandably, is not exhaustive but could be expanded in several areas. One option would be to use an already existing tool for measurement of comorbidity that is organized by organ system, such as the Cumulative Illness Rating Scale.[8] The advantage of such a system is the inclusiveness of a broad range of diagnoses that may impact outcome. The clear disadvantage is the complexity of the system, which would require dedicated time by a knowledgeable medical practitioner to obtain a score. Clearly, this requirement creates significant financial and logistic obstacles for most health care providers and systems trying to limit expenditures. More simplified comorbidity systems such as the Charlson Comorbidity Index[1] may be logistically easier to conduct; however, the breadth of incorporated diagnoses is similar to the existing variables in the current risk stratification system and thus are unlikely to add additional value. Notably, the weighting of variables in the Charlson Comorbidity Index as well as the cumulative scoring of comorbidities is not currently performed in the STS database and could be of some value.

An alternative method would be simply to add in additional variables, which admittedly increases the complexity of data collection. Presently missing disease states for consideration could include functional hepatic disease, states of immunosuppression outside the realm of prednisone use, cognitive impairment, major psychiatric disorders, and substance abuse disorders. Social factors such as living status and states of dependency may be of value as well.

Preoperative functional assessment is clearly of value for the predication of postoperative outcomes. Presently, the STS database uses the Zubrod score as a relative, crude measure of functional status. The Zubrod score, which is very similar to the Eastern Cooperative Oncology Group Performance Status (**Table 1**) and Karnofsky Performance Status are commonly used measures of performance status in oncology. The primary advantage of these measures is the relative ease of obtaining the measurement at a low cost. They have been validated in multiple populations and are well-established in the literature. In contrast, the major disadvantage is the relative subjectivity of the scoring systems. A study looking at Karnofsky Performance Status reveals statistically different results when the score was obtained from the patient, oncologist, and clinic nurse.[9] Not surprisingly, the interobserver variation is less for the Zubrod score owing to the lower degree of granularity in the scoring system.[10] The Zubrod score unfortunately provides little granularity for assessing the elective surgical oncology patient. In the most recent STS Esophageal Cancer Surgery Risk Model, 95.1% of patients included scored a Zubrod score of 0 or 1.[11] It is certainly problematic that an endurance athlete and a patient with severe claudication can be included in the same Zubrod scoring group. Similar challenges exist for the American Society of Anesthesiology Risk classification. In the same Esophageal Cancer Risk Model, 91.5% of patients for elective surgery were included in classes II and III.[11]

More granular assessment tools are certainly available, yet the challenges of subjectivity, complexity of acquisition, and cost create significant obstacles for large-scale, voluntary quality database efforts. Examples of alternative performance measures are listed in **Table 2**. These

Table 1
Zubrod score and ECOG status

Zubrod Score		ECOG Performance Status[18]
0	Asymptomatic	Fully active, able to carry on all predisease performance without restriction
1	Symptomatic	Restricted in physically strenuous activity but ambulatory and able to carry out work of a light or sedentary nature, for example, light house work, office work
2	Symptomatic, <50% in bed during day	Ambulatory and capable of all self-care but unable to carry out any work activities; up and about >50% of waking hours
3	Symptomatic, >50% in bed during day	Capable of only limited self-care; confined to bed or chair >50% of waking hours
4	Bedbound	Completely disabled; cannot carry on any self-care; totally confined to bed or chair
5	Dead	Dead

Abbreviation: ECOG, Eastern Cooperative Oncology Group Performance Status.
From Oken MM, Creech RH, Tormey DC, et al. Toxicity and response criteria of the eastern cooperative oncology group. Am J Clin Oncol 1982;5(6):654; with permission.

measures span a spectrum of complexity from single physical tasks such as grip strength assessment and Timed Get Up and Go to complex questionnaires including 40 to 80 variables with subjective measurement. For large-scale quality efforts, challenges of adopting such measures including cost, uniformity in performance, and reliable performance. Grip strength testing or Timed Get Up and Go are attractive measures that can be done with minimal cost as an additional vital sign to provide an additional facet to the assessment of performance status.

OUTCOME MEASUREMENTS

Selecting appropriate outcome measurements begins with a relatively simple exercise.[12] First answer the question, "What is the intent of the intervention being evaluated?" For lung cancer

Table 2
Performance measure examples

Test	Conduct	Pros	Cons
Timed up and go	Time to stand up from seating, walk 3 m and return to seated position	Easy to perform, minimal cost	Assess single domain
Frailty index	Complex assessment of multiple subjective and objective measures	Comprehensive	Complexlty and cort
SPPB	Performance of several balance and mobility tests	Low cost, easy to perform	Time to complete 5–10 min, assess single domain
Grip strength	Measurement of hand grip strength	Easy and quick to perform	Must purchase dynamometer, measures single domain
EAM	Continuous assessment of actual mobility	Objective measure of function	Costly equipment, validation of monitoring technique

Abbreviations: EAM, electronic activity monitoring; SPPB, Short Physical Performance Battery.
From Kelly CM, Shahrokni A. Moving beyond Karnofsky and ECOG performance status assessments with new technologies. J Oncol 2016;2016:6186543; with permission.

surgery, this would be to cure lung cancer. Not surprisingly, the question that follows is, "How can this be measured?" The Agency for Healthcare Research and Quality has historically used 30-day mortality as a quality endpoint for many medical interventions, including lung cancer surgery. This endpoint satisfies many of the desired characteristics of an ideal outcome. It is objective, easily defined and relatively easy to measure. As Hu and colleagues[13] at the University of Virginia have pointed out, however, it does not fulfill one of the vital requirements, frequency of the event in the population under study.[12] In their review of more than 11,000 lung cancer surgery resections in the Surveillance Epidemiology and End Results database, the mortality rate was 3% to 4%. In the most recent STS Lung Cancer Risk Model, the 30-day mortality rate was 1.4%.[6] The relatively low mortality rates after lung surgery prevents a statistically meaningful analysis of individual centers to differentiate performance. There are various ways, however, to compensate for this.

One solution would be to expand the interval of examination to increase the frequency of events. Hu and colleagues[13] point out that the mortality rate doubles if the period is extended out to 90 days. A similar finding was reported by In and colleagues[14] in the esophagectomy population. In this analysis of the National Cancer Database, the mortality rate after esophagectomy more than doubled from 4.2% at 30 days to 8.9% at 90 days. Clearly, this finding would suggest that the 30-day interval is not providing the complete picture with regard to the ultimate outcome of these major oncologic interventions. In contrast,

the increase may not be entirely attributed to the surgical intervention and could also include the results of adjuvant therapies and unrelated medical events.

An alternative solution to this challenge, is to create composite measures that include surrogate markers for quality to increase the overall event rate. The STS has used this approach to generate statistically meaningful discrimination of contributor performance. For example, the Combined Morbidity and Mortality following Lung Cancer Resection composite score[6] includes postoperative mortality as well as empirically selected morbid events including:

1. Tracheostomy,
2. Reintubation,
3. Initial vent support longer than 48 hours,
4. Adult respiratory distress, syndrome,
5. Bronchopleural fistula
6. Pulmonary embolus,
7. Pneumonia,
8. Unexpected return to the operating room, and
9. Myocardial infarction.

The additional postoperative events were chosen by expert panel agreement. The advantage of this technique is the increased event rate, which permits a useful analysis for comparative audit. In contrast, the choice of specific events could end up introducing a bias that favors certain programs or techniques. An example of this would be the addition of recurrent laryngeal nerve injury to the esophageal composite measure,[11] which would favor those procedures where the anastomosis is performed in the chest and no cervical dissection is performed. Proponents of this addition would argue, however, that the implications of an anastomotic leak in the chest offset this potential bias.

Getting back to the initial exercise, however, the short-term outcome assessments do not truly answer the initial question, "What is the purpose of this intervention?" Clearly, the ideal outcome variable would be the lung cancer cure rate. In 2016, the STS database has added long-term survival data to the registry to address this question. An alternative mechanism, demonstrated by Fernandez and colleagues[15] is the linkage of separate data sources such as the STS Database and Centers for Medicare and Medicaid Services data to provide additional endpoints. A major obstacle to the acquisition of reliable data is the increasingly transient population. Establishing vital status 5 years after an intervention can be quite challenging, especially with the loss of the Social Security Death Index as a useful tool in this regard. In contrast, many cancer programs are mandated by state law to acquire this information thus creating a useful resource for quality programs.

Again, going back to the original question posited at the beginning of this discussion, however, crude mortality rates do not completely answer the question either. Ideally we would like to have progression-free survival (PFS) rates to determine the efficacy of lung cancer resection. The use of PFS, however, creates numerous challenges.[16] One significant challenge is the inherent use of interval censored data. Measurement of progression occurs at intervals after the treatment that need to be defined rigorously. When progression occurs, the event has occurred at some time between the last 2 interval evaluations. If the interval at which it is identified is used as the endpoint, this would provide an overestimation of actual effect. Informative censoring is another challenge of PFS assessment. This censoring occurs when treatment-related toxicity halts the treatment and the patient is no longer followed to determine PFS. Furthermore, simply defining progression can be challenging if treatment interventions are cytostatic. For surgical treatment of lung cancer, this is less of an issue. although confirmation of progression owing to mediastinal lymph node enlargement, for example, may require invasive testing because variability in radiographic interpretation is common. Missing or incomplete data are another obstacle of PFS that can occur owing to loss to follow-up, premature treatment discontinuation, and faulty assessments.[17] Minimizing missing data is essential to the efforts of any quality effort dealing with low incidence events such as mortality after pulmonary resection. Finally, observer bias is of concern and needs to be addressed by independent audit, which can be costly.

SUMMARY

Risk stratification and outcome measurement are 2 essential components of a comparative audit. Rigorous definitions are essential in this process for all included variables. Construction of a functional quality database must balance completeness and accuracy against cost and complexity. Both risk stratification and outcome measurement require a thoughtful approach and continuous maintenance to maintain and effective tool for quality assessment.

REFERENCES

1. Charlson ME, Pompei P, Ales KL, et al. A new method of classifying prognostic comorbidity in longitudinal studies: development and validation. J Chronic Dis 1987;40(5):373–83.
2. Volk ML, Hernandez JC, Lok AS, et al. Modified Charlson comorbidity index for predicting survival after liver transplantation. Liver Transpl 2007; 13(11):1515–20.
3. Quan H, Li B, Couris CM, et al. Updating and validating the Charlson comorbidity index and score for risk adjustment in hospital discharge abstracts using data from 6 countries. Am J Epidemiol 2011; 173(6):676–82.
4. Moonesinghe SR, Mythen MG, Das P, et al. Risk stratification tools for predicting morbidity and mortality in adult patients undergoing major surgery: qualitative systematic review. Anesthesiology 2013; 119(4):959–81.
5. Mak PH, Campbell RC, Irwin MG, et al. The ASA physical status classification: inter-observer consistency. American Society of Anesthesiologists. Anaesth Intensive Care 2002;30(5):633–40.
6. Fernandez FG, Kosinski AS, Burfeind W, et al. The Society of Thoracic Surgeons lung cancer resection risk model: higher quality data and superior outcomes. Ann Thorac Surg 2016;102(2):370–7.
7. Kozower BD, Sheng S, O'Brien SM, et al. STS database risk models: predictors of mortality and major morbidity for lung cancer resection. Ann Thorac Surg 2010;90(3):875–81 [discussion: 881–3].
8. Linn BS, Linn MW, Gurel L. Cumulative illness rating scale. J Am Geriatr Soc 1968;16(5):622–6.
9. Ando M, Ando Y, Hasegawa Y, et al. Prognostic value of performance status assessed by patients themselves, nurses, and oncologists in advanced non-small cell lung cancer. Br J Cancer 2001; 85(11):1634–9.

10. Kelly CM, Shahrokni A. Moving beyond Karnofsky and ECOG performance status assessments with new technologies. J Oncol 2016;2016:6186543.

11. Raymond DP, Seder CW, Wright CD, et al. Predictors of major morbidity or mortality after resection for esophageal cancer: a society of thoracic surgeons general thoracic surgery database risk adjustment model. Ann Thorac Surg 2016;102(1):207–14.

12. Coster WJ. Making the best match: selecting outcome measures for clinical trials and outcome studies. Am J Occup Ther 2013;67(2):162–70.

13. Hu Y, McMurry TL, Wells KM, et al. Postoperative mortality is an inadequate quality indicator for lung cancer resection. Ann Thorac Surg 2014;97(3): 973–9 [discussion: 978–9].

14. In H, Palis BE, Merkow RP, et al. Doubling of 30-day mortality by 90 days after esophagectomy: a critical measure of outcomes for quality improvement. Ann Surg 2016;263(2):286–91.

15. Fernandez FG, Furnary AP, Kosinski AS, et al. Longitudinal follow-up of lung cancer resection from the society of thoracic surgeons general thoracic surgery database in patients 65 years and older. Ann Thorac Surg 2016;101(6):2067–76.

16. Korn HL, Crowley JJ. Overview: progression-free survival as an endpoint in clinical trials with solid tumors. Clin Cancer Res 2013;19(10):2607–12.

17. Sridhara R, Mandrekar SJ, Dodd LE. Missing data and measurement variability in assessing progression-free survival endpoint in randomized clinical trials. Clin Cancer Res 2013;19(10):2613–20.

18. Oken MM, Creech RH, Tormey DC, et al. Toxicity and response criteria of the eastern cooperative oncology group. Am J Clin Oncol 1982;5(6):649–55.

Risk Adjustment and Performance Measurement for Esophageal Cancer Resection

Stephanie G. Worrell, MD[a], Andrew C. Chang, MD[b],*

KEYWORDS

- Esophageal resection • Risk adjustment • Enhanced recovery pathway • Composite score

KEY POINTS

- A straightforward model for predicting outcomes after esophageal resection has proved difficult to identify.
- Prolonged hospital length of stay after esophageal cancer resection has been linked to increased morbidity, mortality, and resource utilization.
- Postoperative complications are associated with a longer length of hospital stay, increased hospital cost, and decreased survival.
- Neither hospital nor provider volume alone can predict outcomes reliably.
- Composite quality measures may provide a benchmark by which outcomes are compared.

INTRODUCTION

Risk adjustment and performance measurements aim to identify a means of achieving high-quality outcomes for patients undergoing esophageal cancer resection. These outcomes are affected by factors related to (1) patients and the disease and (2) the system in which they are treated. Disease-related factors, a patient's health status, and the type of operation influence postoperative complications. Although these factors can be identified in studies, they are not always easily modifiable in an individual patient. System-related factors include surgical team experience and aspects of the health system pertinent to care and treatment of a particular disease. Such elements are the focus for patients, families, and referring physicians deciding how to proceed with health care.

DISEASE-RELATED FACTORS AND RISK ADJUSTMENT

A valid and reliable model for predicting outcomes after esophageal resection has proved difficult to identify, although many models have attempted to address this issue. A recent review article identified more than 10 proposed models, all with similar limitations to clinical application: the lack of high-volume of rare complications and high-quality validation and reproducibility.[1] This review included the Physiological and Operative Severity Score for the enUmeration of Mortality and Morbidity (POSSUM). This model was initially created for risk stratification in general surgery and was found to overpredict mortality in esophageal resection. The POSSUM physiologic score is obtained by a calculation, including the following variables: age, chest radiograph, systolic blood

Disclosure Statement: The authors have nothing to disclose.
[a] Section of Thoracic Surgery, University of Michigan, 1500 East Medical Center Drive, 2120 Taubman Center, Ann Arbor, MI 48109-5344, USA; [b] Section of Thoracic Surgery, Department of Surgery, University of Michigan, 1500 East Medical Center Drive, 2120 Taubman Center, Ann Arbor, MI 48109-5344, USA
* Corresponding author.
E-mail address: andrwchg@med.umich.edu

pressure, heart rate, Glasgow Coma Scale, hemoglobin, white blood cell count, urea, sodium, potassium, and an electrocardiogram. An additional more refined model, the Oesophagogastric POSSUM (O-POSSUM) was developed to address esophageal and gastric surgery.[2] The O-POSSUM model was derived from more than 500 patients undergoing esophageal resections, a majority of which were for malignancy. The O-POSSUM model included the POSSUM physiologic score, cancer stage, urgency of the operation, and type of operation performed. The O-POSSUM score, although cumbersome to calculate, predicted 30-day mortality with an observed-to-expected ratio of 1.03 in the single-level model.[2] This scoring system did not include patients who died in-hospital but after the 30-day time point. Further extending risk stratification by looking at 90-day morbidity and mortality may provide more insight regarding the accuracy of predictive models or other variables that affect long-term outcomes. In a study by Talsma and colleagues[3] looking at the differences in 30-day versus 90-day mortality, there was an increase in mortality from 2.7% to 7% over this time period. Many of these deaths were associated with postoperative complications. Extending follow-up to 1 year, because the 30-day and 90-day benchmarks are not based on statistical endpoints, did not capture many additional operative deaths. Instead, mortality that occurred beyond 90 days was due largely to cancer recurrence rather than immediate complications from the initial operation.[3]

Surgical outcomes are assessed with measurable surrogates, such as length of hospitalization, morbidity, and mortality. Factors in the preoperative, operative, and postoperative periods contribute to the length of hospital stay. It is well established that prolonged hospital length of stay after esophageal cancer resection has been linked to increased morbidity, mortality and resource utilization. Using the National Surgery Quality Improvement Program database, Park and colleagues[4] looked at 3538 esophageal resections and found a median length of hospital stay for all patients of 11 days. The following sections address the factors in preoperative, operative, and postoperative periods that have been shown to affect this length of hospital stay.

Preoperative and Operative Risk

Accurate prognostic models would enhance preoperative risk adjustment and even risk modification but such models have been the most challenging to define. Raymond and colleagues[5] recently published an updated risk model of perioperative morbidity and mortality after esophagectomy for esophageal cancer. This risk assessment is based on more than 4000 patients identified from the Society of Thoracic Surgeons (STS) General Thoracic Surgery Database. The overall perioperative mortality after esophagectomy in this database was 3.1%. With this data set, independent predictors of postoperative morbidity and mortality included age greater than 65 years, the presence of congestive heart failure, Zubrod score greater than 1, past or current smoking status, body mass index greater than 35, squamous histology, and McKeown (or 3-hole) esophagectomy.[5] Other studies also confirm that the procedure associated with the highest rate of prolonged hospitalization is a total esophagectomy with thoracotomy.[4]

Park and colleagues[4] found only 2 independent preoperative predictors of prolonged hospitalization: emergency surgery and modified frailty index. Additionally, Ferguson and Durkin[6] identified 3 preoperative factors that were associated with an increased risk of pulmonary complications: age, spirometry values, and performance status. Other factors identified in the preoperative period to predict those who will have pulmonary complications include history of smoking, cirrhosis, and diabetes.[7–9]

Postoperative Complications

Postoperatively, patients with complications have a longer length of hospital stay. The most common and serious complications after esophageal resection are pulmonary complications. Pulmonary complications occur in more than 20% of patients after esophageal resection.[6,10,11] Law and colleagues[11] found that pulmonary complications were responsible for 55% of hospital deaths after esophageal resection for cancer. In this same study, they identified advanced age, tumor location above the tracheal bifurcation, and operation duration as independent risk factors for pulmonary complications.[11] Other factors independently associated with postoperative pulmonary complications included decreased preoperative pulmonary function test, poor performance status, history of smoking, cirrhosis, and diabetes.[6,7]

Anastomotic leak and renal insufficiency have the highest likelihood of prolonging hospitalization.[4] In addition to a longer length of hospital stay, complications, specifically including anastomotic leak, are associated with increased hospital cost and decreased survival.[12,13] The complications that have been associated with the highest hospital cost are chylothorax requiring reoperation and respiratory failure requiring reintubation.[6] There has been no consistently reported difference in postoperative complications in patients who receive induction chemotherapy and/or radiation (**Table 1**).[11,14]

The difficulty in understanding and comparing studies for postoperative complications is related to the variability in reporting and documentation of complications. A standardized method of reporting may facilitate comparison of outcomes among different reports in the future. Low and colleagues,[15] comprising the Esophagectomy Complications Consensus Group, published a proposed system for defining and recording complications. This group was composed of 21 high-volume esophageal surgeons from 14 countries. Adoption of standardized reporting system may allow for more accurate comparison of patient outcomes and ultimately more accurate predictive models.

SYSTEM-RELATED FACTORS
Enhanced Recovery Pathway

In colorectal surgery, the use of enhanced recovery pathways has been shown to decrease length of hospitalization as well as complication rates.[16] Li and colleagues[17] suggest that the use of enhanced recovery pathways for esophageal resection also is associated with a decreased hospital stay without concomitant increase in complications or readmission rates. The recovery pathway used by Li and colleagues[17] was created from a multidisciplinary care team, including surgery, anesthesiology, nursing, physical therapy, pharmacy, and clinical nutrition. Pathways for the day of surgery through postoperative day 7 were detailed pictorially and posted on the ward. This pathway included no new postoperative interventions from what is routinely done after esophageal

resection; however, they still observed decreased hospital stay. Additional studies using established pathways have shown similar results.[18,19] Low and colleagues[19] used a standard pathway that began within 48 hours of a patient referred to their group for consideration of resection. Implementing the pathway in 340 consecutive patients, they achieved an immediate extubation rate of 99% with 85% of patients walking by postoperative day 1. Furthermore, they reported a mortality rate of less than 1% and an anastomotic leak rate of 3.8%.

The common thread for all reported enhanced recovery pathways in esophageal cancer seems to include a multidisciplinary team dedicated to the care of patients undergoing esophagectomy with the goals of minimizing complications and decreasing length of hospitalization.

Hospital Volume

Hospital volume alone is not a reliable predictor for quality in all procedures, but it has been recognized that many major oncologic operations have better outcomes at higher-volume centers.[20,21] Outcomes based on volume alone also may be skewed due to a patient population that is able to choose where they have their operation. Particularly with esophageal resection, Birkmeyer and colleagues[21] found that more emergency resections occurred at low-volume centers. Therefore, such patients were more likely to be sicker at baseline prior to the operation. After risk adjustment in their analysis, strong correlation persisted between high volume and decreased operative mortality.[21] There was an approximately 12% difference in mortality between the very-high-volume centers performing more than 19 esophagectomies per year and the very-low-volume centers performing fewer than 2 esophagectomies per year.[21] High volume for esophageal resection in Birkmeyer and colleagues' study[21] was defined as 8 to 19 esophagectomies per year, with centers performing more than 19 esophagectomies per year considered very-high-volume centers. Additionally, in a separate study in which high-volume centers were defined as those performing more than 20 esophagectomies per year, van Lanschot and colleagues[22] observed a significant decrease in hospital mortality from 12.1% in low-volume centers to 4.9% in high-volume centers.

More recently, reports from the Leapfrog Group have shown improved outcomes with increased hospital volume for esophageal resection. The Leapfrog Group is a nonprofit organization founded in 2000 by large employers and other purchasers. The group aims to make improvements in

Table 1		
Factors increasing the risk of prolonged hospitalization after esophageal resection		
Preoperative Factors	**Operative Factors**	**Postoperative Factors**
Age >65 y old	Thoracic approach	Anastomotic leak
Congestive heart failure		Respiratory failure
Poor performance status		Chylothorax
Poor pulmonary function tests		
Emergency surgery		
Current or past smoking		

the safety, quality, and affordability of US health through transparency in hospital data. The group reports mortality and hospital volume with major surgical procedures. They have categorized esophagectomy as a high-risk surgery and recommended that patients with esophageal cancer be treated in high-volume centers because of the strong relationship between volumes and outcome for esophagectomy. In contrast with the studies discussed previously, this group defined high-volume centers as those that performed more than 13 esophagectomies per year.[23] In a study using national data from Medicare and the American Hospital Association, of 874 hospitals that perform esophagectomies, more than 90% performed fewer than 3 esophagectomies per year.[24]

Although hospital volume likely is a surrogate for quality of care, other investigators have shown that this metric alone is not a precise or accurate way to predict outcomes.[25,26] Composite measures that address process and provider volume may identify further opportunities for quality improvement.

COMPOSITE MEASURES

The STS has developed composite quality measures for both cardiac surgery procedures and lobectomy for lung cancer.[27,28] A recent publication from the STS General Thoracic Surgery Database Task Force by[29] created a composite score using operative mortality and major postoperative events or complications reported to the STS General Thoracic Surgery Database as a quality measure for outcomes after esophageal resection for cancer. This study included 4321 patients who underwent esophagectomy for esophageal cancer by 167 database participants. The 30-day operative mortality was 3.1% with 33% of patients experiencing at least 1 major complication. The reliability of the composite score increased to 58% with a participant operative volume minimum of 5 cases performed per year with no significant increase in reliability compared with the highest-volume groups, performing greater than 20 esophagectomies per year.[29] The composite score was calculated by the same methodology used for other STS composite scores[27,28] and was derived by the weighted sum of a mortality score and a major complication score. Mortality and major complications scores were weighted inversely by their respective standard deviations across participants and then normalized by the sum of inverses of these standard deviations. The types of complications included unexpected return to the operating room, anastomotic leak requiring medical or surgical treatment, reintubation, initial ventilator support greater than 48 hours, pneumonia, renal failure, and recurrent laryngeal nerve injury.[29]

Each eligible participant in the STS General Thoracic Surgery Database was assigned a risk-adjusted composite score. Based on a comparison of the mean STS score to each participant's derived composite score, the participants were assigned into 1 of 3 performance categories. The categories were defined as 1 star, for a lower-than-expected composite score; 2 star, for a composite score that fell within the 95% credible interval for the STS cohort mean composite score; or 3 star, for a higher-than-expected composite score.[29] Of 5 3-star participants identified by this methodology, 1 is considered lower volume, although still with an average esophagectomy volume of 5 or more per year.

This composite score, based on a prospectively maintained database, may prove more accurate and reliable than current simple composite scores derived from administrative databases. Additionally, a composite score is more reliable than a simple measure of mortality due to the low event rate. Of the 167 participants reporting data for esophagectomy, 70 participants reported sufficient operative volume, that is, 15 esophagectomies (5 per year) during the 3-year study period to receive a reliable composite score. It remains unclear whether refinements to this model can improve the reliability such that lower volume participants can receive a composite score.

SUMMARY

To ensure quality care, it is vitally important for surgeons to identify in the preoperative setting those patients at highest risk. One single model to predict all patient outcomes has yet to be identified. The O-POSSUM model may be the most accurate model to date. The use of enhanced recovery pathways also can improve patient outcomes by including a multidisciplinary team dedicated to the care of patients undergoing esophageal resection with the goal of minimizing complications and decreasing length of hospitalization. Newer composite quality measures may provide a benchmark by which outcomes can be monitored for quality improvement. Continued evaluation and re-evaluation of personal and institutional outcomes may elucidate areas for improvement ultimately resulting in better patient survival and greater quality of life.

REFERENCES

1. Warnell I, Chincholkar M, Eccles M. Predicting perioperative mortality after oesophagectomy: a

systematic review of performance and methods of multivariate models. Br J Anaesth 2015;114(1): 34–43.

2. Tekkis PP, McCulloch P, Poloniecki DR, et al. Risk-adjusted prediction of operative mortality in oesophagogastric surgery with O-POSSUM. Br J Surg 2004;91:288–95.

3. Talsma AK, Lingsma HF, Steyerberg EW, et al. The 30-day versus in-hospital and 90-day mortality after esophagectomy as indicators for quality of care. Ann Surg 2014;260(2):267–73.

4. Park KU, Rubinfeld I, Hodari A, et al. Prolonged length of stay after esophageal resection: identifying drivers of increased length of stay using the NSQIP database. J Am Coll Surg 2016; 223(2):286–90.

5. Raymond DP, Seder CW, Wright CD, et al. Predictors of major morbidity or mortality after resection for esophageal cancer: A Society of Thoracic Surgeons General Thoracic Surgery Database risk adjustment model. Ann Thorac Surg 2016;102(1): 207–14.

6. Fergerson MK, Durkin AE. Preoperative predication of the risk of pulmonary complications after esophagectomy for cancer. J Thorac Cardiovasc Surg 2002;123(4):661–9.

7. Karl RC, Schreiber R, Boulware D, et al. Factors affecting morbidity, mortality, and survival in patients undergoing Ivor Lewis esophagogastrectomy. Ann Surg 2000;231:635–43.

8. Wright CD, Kucharczuk JC, O'Brien SM, et al. Predictors of major morbidity and mortality after esophagectomy for esophageal cancer: a Society of Thoracic Surgeons General Thoracic Surgery Database risk adjustment model. J Thorac Cardiovasc Surg 2009;137(3):587–96.

9. Dhungel B, Diggs BS, Hunter JG, et al. Patient and peri-operative predictors of morbidity and mortality after esophagectomy: American College of Surgeons National Surgical Quality Improvement Program (ACS-NSQIP), 2005–2008. J Gastrointest Surg 2010;14(10):1492–501.

10. Bailey SH, Bull DA, Harpole DH, et al. Outcomes after esophagectomy: a ten-year prospective cohort. Ann Thorac Surg 2003;75:217–22.

11. Law S, Wong K, Kwok K, et al. Predictive factors for postoperative pulmonary complications and mortality after esophagectomy for cancer. Ann Surg 2004; 240(5):791–800.

12. Carrott PW, Markar SR, Kuppusamy MK, et al. Accordion Severity Grading System: assessment of relationship between costs, length of hospital stay, and survival in patients with complications after esophagectomy for cancer. J Am Coll Surg 2012; 215(3):331–6.

13. Rizk NP, Bach PB, Schrag D, et al. The impact of complications on outcomes after resection for esophageal and gastroesophageal junction carcinoma. J Am Coll Surg 2004;198:42–50.

14. Doty JR, Salazar JD, Forastiere AA, et al. Postesophagectomy morbidity, mortality, and length of hospital stay after preoperative chemoradiation therapy. Ann Thorac Surg 2002;74:227–31.

15. Low DE, Alderson D, Cecconello I, et al. International consensus on standardization of data collection for complications associated with esophagectomy: Esophagectomy Complications Consensus Group. Ann Surg 2015;262:286–94.

16. Muller S, Zalunardo MP, Hubner M, et al. A fast-track program reduces complications and length of hospital stay after open colonic surgery. Gastroenterology 2009;136(3):842–7.

17. Li C, Ferri LE, Mulder DS, et al. An enhanced recovery pathway decreases duration of stay after esophagectomy. Surgery 2012;152(4):606–14.

18. Munitiz V, Martinez-de-Haro LF, Ortiz A, et al. Effectiveness of a written clinical pathway for enhanced recovery after transthoracic (Ivor Lewis) oesophagectomy. Br J Surg 2010;97:714–8.

19. Low DE, Kunz S, Schembre D, et al. Esophagectomy–it's not just about mortality anymore: standardized perioperative clinical pathways improve outcomes in patients with esophageal cancer. J Gastrointest Surg 2007;11:1395–402.

20. Begg CB, Cramer LD, Hoskins WJ, et al. Impact of hospital volume on operative mortality for major cancer surgery. JAMA 1998;280:1747–51.

21. Birkmeyer JD, Siewers AE, Finlayson EV, et al. Hospital volume and surgical mortality in the United States. N Engl J Med 2002;246:1128–37.

22. van Lanschot JJ, Julscher JB, Buskens CJ, et al. Hospital volume and hospital mortality for esophagectomy. Cancer 2001;91(8):1574–8.

23. Birkmeyer JD, Dimick JB. Potential benefits of the new Leapfrog standards: effect of process and outcomes measures. Surgery 2004;135:569–75.

24. Funk LM, Gawande AA, Semel ME, et al. Esophagectomy outcomes at low-volume hospitals: the association between systems characteristics and mortality. Ann Surg 2011 May;253(5):912–7.

25. Kozower BD, Stukenborg GJ. The relationship between hospital lung cancer resection volume and patient mortality risk. Ann Surg 2011;254(6): 1032–7.

26. Cooke CR, Kennedy EH, Wiitala WL, et al. Despite variation in volume, Veterans Affairs hospitals show consistent outcomes among patients with non-postoperative mechanical ventilation. Crit Care Med 2012;40(9):2569–75.

27. Kozower BD, O'Brien SM, Kosinski AS, et al. The Society of Thoracic Surgeons composite score for rating program performance for lobectomy for lung cancer. Ann Thorac Surg 2016;101(4): 1379–86.

28. Shahian DM, He X, Jabobs JP, et al. The Society of Thoracic Surgeons composite measure of individual surgeon performance for adult cardiac surgery: a report of The Society of Thoracic Surgeons Quality Measurement Task Force. Ann Thorac Surg 2015;100(4):1315–24.

29. The Society of Thoracic Surgeons General Thoracic Surgery Database Task Force. The Society of Thoracic Surgeons composite score for evaluating esophagectomy for esophageal cancer. Ann Thorac Surg 2017;103(5):1661–7.

Oncologic Quality Indicators in Thoracic Surgery

Jessica Hudson, MD, MSc[a], Tara Semenkovich, MD[a],
Varun Puri, MD, MSCI[b,*]

KEYWORDS

- Quality • Lung cancer • Esophageal cancer • Staging • R0 resection • Lymphadenectomy
- Multidisciplinary treatment

KEY POINTS

- Quality of care can be evaluated through structure, process, and outcome measures.
- Adherence to evidence-based quality metrics improves patient survival outcomes.
- Strongly supported quality measures for lung cancer include preoperative mediastinal staging, timely anatomic resection via a minimally invasive approach, complete (R0) resection, adequate lymph node sampling, multidisciplinary care teams, and clinical care pathways.
- Strongly supported quality measures for esophageal cancer include staging with PET-computed tomography and endoscopic ultrasound, achieving an R0 resection, performing an adequate lymphadenectomy, and administering induction chemoradiation for locally advanced disease.

INTRODUCTION

Quality in surgical care is notoriously difficult to define, but a thorough discussion of quality indicators rests on an understanding of this concept, as well as an organized structure in which to consider multiple aspects of the care provided. Oncologic quality is essentially an assessment of the value of the various aspects of medical care provided to a patient from their first contact with a physician through completion of their care, with a goal of treatment or cure of disease, prolongation of survival, palliation of suffering, improvement in quality of life, or achievement of other aims important to the patient or society.

Donabedian[1] outlined a central framework in which the quality of medical care could be analyzed, focusing specifically on the patient-provider interaction. This model divides the assessment of quality into 3 categories: structure, process, and outcome measures (**Fig. 1**). These classifications of quality indicators build on each other and can be fragmented further to allow for a detailed analysis of the entire course of patient care.

Structure measures are defined as the characteristics of the environment and the medical providers that account for the overall setting in which care is provided. These metrics focus on the most physical aspects of care: hospitals, operating suites, instruments, and technology, as well as the experience-related aspects of care: training of surgeons and staff, availability of multiple medical specialties, volume, and centralization of care. The philosophy behind assessing these measures is that optimization of the setting will facilitate the provision of ideal medical care. Certain structure measures will be discussed later within this volume, so an in-depth discussion will be deferred here.

Disclosure Statement: The authors have no relevant disclosures.
[a] Department of Cardiothoracic Surgery, Washington University School of Medicine, 660 South Euclid Avenue, Campus Box 8109, St Louis, MO 63110, USA; [b] Department of Cardiothoracic Surgery, Washington University School of Medicine, 660 South Euclid Avenue, Campus Box 8234, St Louis, MO 63110, USA
* Corresponding author.
E-mail address: puriv@wudosis.wustl.edu

Thorac Surg Clin 27 (2017) 227–244
http://dx.doi.org/10.1016/j.thorsurg.2017.04.001

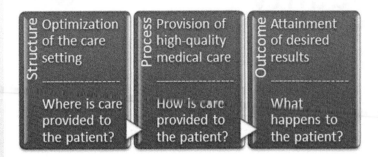

Fig. 1. A model for understanding quality of care in medicine as proposed by Donabedian. The 3 categories outlined provide a framework for discussion. (*Data from* Donabedian A. Evaluating the quality of medical care. Milbank Mem Fund Q 1966;33(4):691–729.)

Process measures are defined as evaluations of how care is provided to the patient in the setting previously described. These measures look at diagnostics, patient selection for appropriate care, and the treatments or interventions provided. Assessing these measures allows one to determine if high-quality care has been provided to the patient. This is based on the idea that patients receiving complete application of evidence-based medicine will have better outcomes. Process measures are of particular interest because these identify specific points in the patient's treatment in which practice could potentially be changed to enhance the patient's eventual outcome.

Outcome measures are defined as metrics, tracking the results of the entire medical process that the patient experiences. Outcomes are typically the most easily comprehensible of the 3 types of measures because they often track the discrete events that are easily identifiable and able to be precisely quantified. This category includes measures such as survival, cancer recurrence, and treatment-related complications. These outcome measures are susceptible to effects of factors other than simply the care provided. In the Donabedian framework, variables are often closely linked. Examples of these measures can be seen in (**Fig. 2**). A subset of outcomes measures is now of national interest and tracked by multiple entities. Organizations, such as the American College of Chest Physicians (ACCP), the British Thoracic Society (BTS), the European Society of Thoracic Surgeons (ESTS), the American College of Surgeons (ACS), the National Comprehensive Cancer Network (NCCN), and the Society of Thoracic Surgeons (STS), have proposed, and intermittently updated, treatment guidelines aimed at improving the quality, effectiveness, and efficiency of cancer care worldwide. These guidelines often represent a combination of best available evidence and expert opinion.

With a special focus on process and outcome measures, this framework is used to evaluate quality indicators currently relevant in thoracic surgical oncology in the preoperative, intraoperative, and postoperative phases. Current quality measures for lung and esophageal cancer are explored, and the relevant evidence and guidelines supporting use of these quality measures is discussed.

ONCOLOGIC QUALITY INDICATORS IN SURGICALLY RESECTABLE NON-SMALL CELL LUNG CANCER

Innumerable quality process indicators for non-small cell lung cancer (NSCLC) have been reported in the literature. Recently, a multidisciplinary expert panel used a modified Delphi process and concluded that, although mortality, morbidity, survival, and length of stay were the most important outcomes indicators, they were insufficient metrics of quality oncologic care delivery. Instead, they recommended 12 evidence-based and 5 consensus-based processes and outcome measures related to preoperative assessment, pathologic staging and evaluation, surgical resection, and adjuvant therapy.[2] Subsequently, Numan and colleagues[3,4] used the Donabedian framework for 2 systematic reviews to identify supported indicators for quality preoperative and postoperative care for stage I-IIIA NSCLC. Both strategies identified factors such as hospital size or teaching status, surgeon specialty, and access to multidisciplinary care teams as significant contributors to favorable oncologic outcomes.[3] Surgeon or hospital procedural volume was not clearly related to postoperative mortality (see Benjamin D. Kozower and George J. Stukenborg's article, "Volume Outcome Relationships in Thoracic Surgery," in this issue for further discussion). Because this article focuses on measures that lend themselves to easier targeted intervention, these structural measures are not addressed further. Instead, the actionable process measures that are strongly linked to patient outcomes have been coalesced into 9 divisions, addressing each evidence-based element in turn, as well touching on important issues of clinical equipoise. The

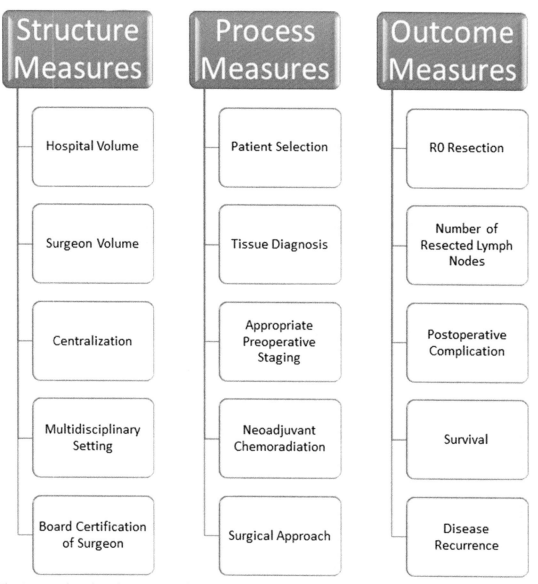

Fig. 2. Examples of quality measures for thoracic cancers. (*Data from* Courrech Staal EFW, Wouters MWJM, Boot H, et al. Quality-of-care indicators for esophageal cancer surgery: A review. Eur J Surg Oncol 2010;36(11): 1035–43.)

discussion about improving survival in lung cancer is further framed by the preoperative, intraoperative, and postoperative points of intervention (**Fig. 3**).

Preoperative Quality Measures in Clinical Stage I-IIIA Lung Cancer

Preoperative quality measures are intended to ensure accurate diagnoses, adequate staging, and efficient care delivery. **Table 1** summarizes the current evidence-based preoperative process

quality measures. This discussion focuses on 3 specific measures: preoperative mediastinal staging, tissue diagnosis, and early surgical resection.

In patients with suspected NSCLC, adequate patient management is contingent on accurate oncologic staging. However, data suggest that it is poorly done.[5,13,14] When disease is localized to the chest, accurate preoperative mediastinal staging is critical.[5,14,15] Several observational studies have shown improved staging accuracy with the utilization of complementary techniques.[16,17] Farjah and colleagues[18] retrospectively assessed

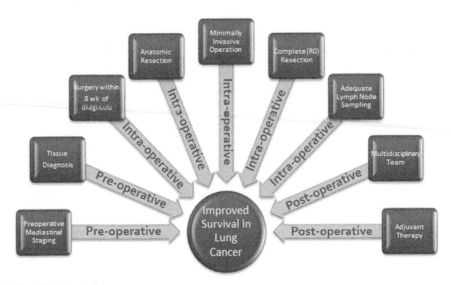

Fig. 3. Quality indicators in lung cancer.

the benefit of multimodality mediastinal staging for stage I-III NSCLC and found that patients who underwent bimodality staging tests (computed tomography [CT] plus PET or CT plus invasive tissue sampling) or trimodality staging tests (CT, PET, and invasive staging) had significantly lower risk of death, even when adjusted for stage (hazard ratio [HR] 0.58 [0.56–0.60] for bimodality and HR 0.49 [0.45–.054] for trimodality). However, 2 underpowered randomized controlled trials showed no benefit of CT plus PET on diagnostic accuracy, cost savings, or survival.[19,20] In the absence of higher level evidence, quality mediastinal staging entails bimodal preoperative imaging. Note that the influence of PET on treatment delays remains under debate.

Patients with peripheral, clinical stage I NSCLC without concerning PET findings can be considered adequately staged. With extensive mediastinal infiltration, definitive invasive mediastinal staging is indicated.[15] Generally speaking, rigid bronchoscopy with washings, brushes, and forceps biopsies (FBs) are insufficiently sensitive (43%–57%), though they can be improved when combined with fluoroscopy for peripheral lesions. The diagnostic yield of FB is 50.5% to 81.5%, which is further improved with cytopathologic examination.[4] In both visible and nonvisible tumors, transbronchial or ultrasound-guided fine needle aspirations increase the diagnostic yield approximately 20% compared with bronchoscopy with FB.[4,5] The sensitivities and specificities of most image-guided techniques are similar, but the false-negative rate is higher for needle aspirations than for mediastinoscopy (**Table 2**). High negative predictive values often necessitate confirmatory

testing.[4,5,15] Emerging data support the complementary roles of endoscopic ultrasound (EUS) with needle aspiration (NA), endobronchial ultrasound (EBUS) with NA, and mediastinoscopy to avoid futile surgery.[4,15,21] In conclusion, there is high level evidence to support PET-CT, endosonography, and the combination of histologic and cytologic pathologic examination for quality oncologic staging of the mediastinum.[4,5]

Diagnosis at an earlier stage and screening of high-risk individuals are known to improve patient survival.[22] However, the median time from diagnosis to treatment of NSCLC has increased over the last decade.[23] Although patient-specific factors influence treatment delays, even when adjusted for higher risk characteristics, surgical resection greater than 8 weeks from diagnosis is independently associated with pathologic upstaging and decreased median survival, yet nearly 20% of patients experience significant care delay.[6] This is particularly alarming for socioeconomically disadvantaged patients who already suffer from disparities in treatment and outcomes for NSCLC.[24,25] Ensuring quality care via timely surgical resection requires acknowledgment of disease-specific, systemic, and cultural barriers to meeting this metric.

Intraoperative Quality Measures in Clinical Stage I-IIIA Lung Cancer

Intraoperative quality measures are designed to balance maximizing oncologic benefit while minimizing the risk of serious surgical complications. **Tables 3** and **4** summarize the current evidence-based intraoperative process quality measures,

Table 1
Preoperative quality measures in clinical stage I-IIIA non-small cell lung cancer

Category	Quality Metric	Recommended by	Evidence Grade
Bronchoscopy	Unless obstructing lesion, preferably performed during planned resection	BTS NCCN	2A
Clinical staging	Clarified and recorded before surgery	BTS STS	—
Diagnostics	Pulmonary function testing and electrocardiogram Further physiologic testing as clinically indicated	ACCP BTS NCCN Darling et al.	2A
Imaging	Contrast CT of chest and upper abdomen including adrenals FDG-PET skull base to knees or whole body If stage IIB-III, contrast brain MRI	BTS NCCN Darling et al. Numan et al.	2A
Neoadjuvant therapy, N0-N1 disease	Not recommended	ACCP NCCN Numan et al.	1A-1C
Neoadjuvant therapy, discrete N2 disease	Surgery is not the first course of treatment with discrete N2 disease Give either definitive chemoradiation or induction therapy followed by surgery	ACCP NCCN Numan et al.	1A-1C
Prophylactic cranial irradiation	Not recommended outside of a clinical trial if complete response after concurrent chemoradiotherapy	ACCP	2C
Radiotherapy	Consider in stage III to increase mediastinal downstaging	Numan et al.	2B
Radiotherapy, definitive	Do not give only radiotherapy if good performance status Preferable to no therapy if unable to tolerate subanatomic resection In stage III, may increase mediastinal downstaging	ACCP BTS Numan et al.	1A-1C
Restaging	Repeat CT/PET after induction therapy to exclude disease progression	NCCN Numan et al.	2A
Timing of surgery	Surgery within 8 wk of diagnosis Caveat: If neoadjuvant therapies are indicated, they should be within 4 mo preoperatively	ACCP Reifel et al. Samson et al.	—
Tissue diagnosis	Should obtain before anatomic resection Select least invasive biopsy with highest yield If strong clinical suspicion, specimen not needed preoperatively	ACCP BTS NCCN Numan et al.	1C-2A
Treatment planning	Surgical resection unless contraindicated	ACCP BTS Darling et al. Numan et al.	1B

Abbreviation: CT, computed tomography.
Data from Refs.[2–12,66]

specific to clinical stage. This discussion focuses on 4 specific measures: anatomic resection, complete (R0) resection, minimally invasive operations, and adequate lymph node (LN) sampling (see **Fig. 3**).

Although some nuances remain, R0 anatomic resection, when feasible, is considered the standard of care.[2,3,7,8,28] Similarly, minimally invasive approaches should be undertaken when feasible

Table 2
Techniques for mediastinal staging, in order of increased invasiveness of technique, with available associated performance metrics

Diagnostic Modality	Sensitivity, Mean (Range), %	Specificity, Mean (Range), %	False Negatives, Mean (Range), %	False Positives, Mean (Range), %
EUS-NA	84 (45–100)	99.5 (88–100)	19 (0–32)	0.4 (0–7)
TBNA	78 (14–100)	100 (96–100)	28 (0–66)	0 (0–11)
EBUS-NA	90 (79–95)	100	24 (1–37)	0
TTNA	90 (72–100)	100	0	0
VATS staging	— (37–100)	100	15 (0–58)	0
Mediastinoscopy	80 (40–97)	100	10 (3–20)	0

Abbreviations: EBUS-NA, endobronchial ultrasound with needle aspiration; EUS-NA, endoscopic ultrasound with needle aspiration; TBNA, transbronchial needle aspiration; TTNA, transthoracic needle aspiration; VATS, video-assisted thoracoscopic surgery.

Data from Detterbeck FC, Lewis SZ, Diekemper R, et al. Executive Summary: Diagnosis and management of lung cancer, 3rd edition: American College of Chest Physicians evidence-based clinical practice guidelines. Chest 2013;143(5):7S–37S.

Table 3
Intraoperative quality measures in clinical stage I-IIIA non-small cell lung cancer

Category	Quality Metric	Recommended by	Evidence Grade
Anatomic Resection	Lobectomy, if feasible, otherwise: anatomic sublobar resection, margins > maximal tumor diameter or 2 cm for larger tumors	ACCP BTS NCCN Darling et al. Numan et al.	1B, 1C
Anatomic Resection	R0 sleeve or bronchoplastic resection preferable to pneumonectomy	ACCP NCCN Darling et al. Numan et al.	2C
Anatomic Resection	Sublobar resection with negative margins in predominantly ground glass opacity lesions <2 cm	ACCP	2C
Complete Resection	R0 resection	ACCP NCCN Darling et al. Numan et al.	1A
Mediastinal Assessment	At least 10 nodes are removed and examined	ACS Commission on Cancer Darling et al.	2A
Mediastinal Assessment	Minimum sampling of 3 mediastinal nodal stations (Right: 2R, 4R, 7, 8, 9 Left: 4L, 5, 6, 7, 8, 9)	ESTS NCCN Darling et al.	2A
Mediastinal Assessment	Systematic mediastinal lymph node sampling or dissection at time of resection	ACCP ESTS NCCN Darling et al.	1B
Minimally Invasive Operation	Video-assisted thoracoscopic surgery approach when feasible	ACCP NCCN Numan et al.	2C
Tissue diagnosis	If not definitive preoperative, must obtain intraoperatively before anatomic resection	ESTS NCCN	2A

Data from Refs.[2–4,7–9,26,27]

Table 4
Intraoperative quality measures specific to clinical stage IIIA (N2-N3, M0) non-small cell lung cancer

Category	Quality Metric	Recommended by	Evidence Grade
Anatomic resection	Pneumonectomy is ill-advised after neoadjuvant therapy	NCCN	2A
Mediastinal assessment if confirming suspected N2 disease	Abort operation	ACCP	2C
Mediastinal assessment if find occult N2 disease	If complete resection of primary tumor is feasible, perform mediastinal lymph node dissection or systematic sampling	ACCP	2C

Data from NCCN Clinical Practice Guidelines in Oncology: Non-small cell lung cancer (National Comprehensive Cancer Network). 2017. Available at: https://www.nccn.org/professionals/physician_gls/pdf/nscl.pdf. Accessed March 29, 2017; and Ramnath N, Dilling TJ, Harris LJ, et al. Treatment of Stage III Non-small Cell Lung Cancer Chest 2013;143(5):e314S–40S.

because they correlate with shorter length of stay and improved pain control, though result in more variable performance of LN assessment despite similar overall survival.[4,7,28,29] Pathologic examination of higher numbers of LNs is associated with increased disease-free and overall survival but the definition of adequate LN staging has been more nebulous.[30] The Commission on Cancer recommends pathologic examination of at least 10 LNs, whereas the NCCN encourages sampling from 3 mediastinal nodal stations (see **Table 3**).[26] When compared with systematic sampling, lymphadenectomy or LN dissection for stage I-IIIA NSCLC identified more N2 disease but was not associated with improved survival. Therefore, systematic sampling is likely sufficient.[3,31]

Samson and colleagues[32] explored adherence to quality measures in stage I NSCLC resection using the National Cancer Database, with special attention to anatomic resection, R0 resection, sampling of 10 or more LNs, and surgery within 8 weeks of diagnosis. They reported that adherence to an increased number of quality metrics was associated with statistically significant higher rates of pathologic upstaging but also improved overall survival. As it pertains to LN sampling, a slight temporal trend was noted, yet only 34% of patients in 2013 had more than 10 LNs sampled. Thus, real-world compliance remains suboptimal.

Postoperative Quality Measures in Clinical Stage I-IIIA Lung Cancer

Postoperative quality measures are designed to optimize adjuvant therapy and disease surveillance while minimizing unnecessary risks and costs. Therefore, metrics vary based on pathologic stage. **Tables 5** and **6** summarize the current

evidence-based postoperative process quality measures for stage I-II and stage IIIA NSCLC, respectively.

The nuances of adjuvant therapy are beyond the scope of this discussion but are stratified by the current recommendations based on pathologic stage and adequacy of surgical resection. Pathologic microscopic invasion of the bronchial stump (R1) has a significantly worse prognosis, with 1-year and 5-year survival rates between 20% to 50% and 0% to 20%, respectively.[35,36] Because peribronchial residual disease is associated with metastatic LN involvement and functional limitations, subsequent treatment, including reresection, remains controversial (see **Table 5**).[4,7,9,15]

There is high-level evidence to support multidisciplinary oncology care teams. Within a multidisciplinary care model for NSCLC, Numan and colleagues[4] elucidated the novel process quality measure of clinical care. The elements of such standardized care pathways can be seen in **Table 7** and correlate with decreased length of stay, fewer pulmonary complications, and improved pain control. Specifically, several randomized controlled trials demonstrated improved pain control with preemptive epidural analgesia or nerve block and decreased air leaks with chest tubes managed on water seal.[3] Implementation of a clinical care pathway for NSCLC can lead to widespread improved performance on quality metrics.[37]

ONCOLOGIC QUALITY INDICATORS IN SURGICALLY RESECTABLE ESOPHAGEAL CANCER

As in lung cancer, there are several important recommended process and outcome quality metrics for esophageal cancer.

Table 5
Postoperative quality measures specific to clinical stage I-II non-small cell lung cancer

Category	Subcategory	Quality Metric	Recommended by	Evidence Grade
Adjuvant chemotherapy	R0 in stage IA	Not currently recommended	ACCP BTS Numan et al.	1B
Adjuvant chemotherapy	R0 in stage IB	Controversial	ACCP BTS Numan et al.	2C
Adjuvant chemotherapy	R0 in stage IIA or IIB	Platinum-based chemotherapy	ACCP BTS Numan et al.	1A
Radiotherapy	R0 in stage II	Not currently recommended	ACCP Burdett et al,[34] 2016 Numan et al.	2A
Radiotherapy	R1 resection in stage I or II	Controversial	ACCP Numan et al.	2C
Positive margins (R1 and R2)	Pathologic stage IA	Reresection (preferred) or radiotherapy	NCCN	2A
Positive margins (R1 and R2)	Pathologic stage IB-IIB	Reresection (preferred) with or without adjuvant therapy	NCCN	2A

Data from Refs.[4,7–9,34]

Evidence that Quality Matters for Patient Survival

A recent review by Courrech Staal and colleagues[38] explored the published evidence behind a very wide range of quality metrics that have been suggested in esophageal cancer operations using the Donabedian framework of structure, process, and outcome measures. With regard to structural measures that affected postoperative mortality, the investigators found there was strong or considerable evidence for high-volume hospitals and surgeons, as well as surgeons with thoracic specialty training. Within the process measures, they found that patient selection (which was captured in their review as age and functional status), staging, and neoadjuvant chemoradiation affected patient survival. Of the outcome measures assessed, they noted substantial evidence supporting improved survival in R0 resections, patients with higher nodal counts, and those who escaped postoperative complications. This review nicely outlines the overall level of support behind various quality metrics.

Several studies have examined discretely the effect that adherence to sets of quality measures can have on patient survival in esophageal cancer. Recently, Samson and colleagues[39] evaluated the survival implications in National Cancer Database subjects of achieving an R0 resection, performing a lymphadenectomy of 15 or more

Table 6
Postoperative quality measures specific to clinical stage IIIA (N2-N3, M0) non-small cell lung cancer

Category	Quality Metric	Recommended by	Evidence Grade
Adjuvant chemo-radiotherapy	Concurrent combination platinum-based chemotherapy and radiotherapy, tailored to performance, nodal status, and completeness of resection	ACCP BTS NCCN	1A-2C
Positive margins (R1 and R2)	No re-resection Give planned adjuvant chemoradiotherapy	NCCN	2A

Data from Refs.[7,8,11]

Table 7
Postoperative quality measures in clinical stage I-IIIA non-small cell lung cancer

Category	Quality Metric	Recommended by	Evidence Grade
Fast track or care pathway	Introduce a clinical care pathway emphasizing management of (1) pain, (2) chest tube, (3) mobilization, (4) nutrition, (5) intravenous infusion, (6) oxygen support, (7)wound care, (8) patient education, (9) discharge, and (10) aspiration prevention	Numan et al.	2A-2B
Surveillance after definitive therapy	Serial chest CT No routine PET or brain MRI	NCCN	2A
Timely adjuvant chemotherapy	Systemic chemotherapy is given within 6 mo postoperatively	ACCP	2B
Timely hospital discharge	Prolonged postoperative hospital course after elective lobectomy for lung cancer is defined as >14 d (risk adjusted by STS)	STS Darling et al. Numan et al.	—

Data from Refs.[2,3,7,9,11,33]

nodes, and using induction treatment of locally advanced cancer. This study found a temporal trend toward increasing attainment of more quality metrics, and demonstrated a reduction in mortality corresponding to the number of measures achieved. Additionally, meeting all selected quality measures decreased the mortality HR to 0.21 (0.14–0.32) for early stage cancer and to 0.54 (0.40–0.73) for locally advanced cancer. A summary of the observed improvement in median survival for both early and locally advanced esophageal cancer based on quality measures can be found in **Table 8**.

The effect of a quality score in a single-institution cohort of locally advanced subjects with esophageal cancer was examined by Molena and colleagues[40] In this study, a score was generated by examining 7 quality indicators based on NCCN guidelines: histologic classification,

tumor location, tumor grade, surgery, induction chemoradiation, staging with PET-CT and EUS, and 2 restaging scans. Subject outcomes were compared between 2 groups, those above (high quality care) and those below (low quality care) the median score. The investigators again found an improvement in survival of an additional 6 months for those subjects receiving higher quality care, with a HR of 0.58 (0.37–0.90).

Selected Quality Measures

These studies demonstrate an improvement in patient survival with adherence to quality guidelines but also demonstrate the variation in definition of quality metrics. This article discusses the evidence behind 4 of the most widely used process and outcome quality measures in esophageal cancer: staging with PET-CT and EUS, achieving an

Table 8
Survival based on number of quality measures met: including complete resection, lymphadenectomy of at least 15 nodes, and induction therapy for locally advanced disease

Number of Quality Measures Met	Early Stage		Locally Advanced	
	Median Survival (mo)	Percentage of Patients, %	Median Survival (mo)	Percentage of Patients, %
0	23.7 ± 3.6	70.1	14.4 ± 2.4	1.5
1	104 ± 4.9		19.5 ± 0.9	10.5
2	123 ± 12.6	29.9	31.1 ± 0.8	55.9
3	NA (no induction treatment)		36.1 ± 1.8	32.1

Data from Samson P, Puri V, Broderick S, et al. Adhering to quality measures in esophagectomy is associated with improved survival in all stages of esophageal cancer. Ann Thorac Surg 2017;103(4):1101–8.

R0 resection, performing an adequate lymphade-nectomy, and administering induction chemora-diation for locally advanced esophageal cancer (**Fig. 4**).

Staging with PET-Computed Tomography and Endoscopic Ultrasound

Following diagnosis with endoscopy and biopsy, staging in esophageal cancer should include PET and CT to assess for regional and distant spread, and, if no metastatic disease is noted, EUS should be used to assess the extent of local and regional disease. PET and CT should be performed to eval-uate for regional and distant spread, and repeated following induction therapy to reassess resect-ability. A summary of studies supporting the use of these staging modalities can be reviewed in **Table 9**.

EUS use is recommended for routine staging when there is no evidence of distant metastases because of its utility in locoregional staging. This is supported by a large meta-analysis[42] that pooled 49 studies to include more than 2500 sub-jects. The findings were that EUS is sensitive and specific for both tumor (T) and node (N) staging, with the following sensitivities and specificities, respectively, by stage: T1: 82%, 99%; T2: 81%, 96%; T3: 91%, 94%; T4: 92%, 97%; and N: 85%, 85%. EUS performs better than PET or CT for local and regional staging because of the ability to distinguish layers of the esophageal wall for tu-mor staging and examine periesophageal stations of mediastinal LNs for nodal staging. One meta-analysis[43] compared all 3 staging modalities and confirmed that EUS is the most sensitive for detec-tion of nodal metastasis (80% vs 50%–57%) but less specific than PET or CT (70% vs 83%–85%). Another systematic review[41] on PET scanning in esophageal cancer found the imaging to be most helpful for detecting distant metastases (sensitivity 67% and specificity 97%).

STS Guidelines on Staging[44] and NCCN Guide-lines[45] recommend that for both early and locally advanced esophageal cancer, staging should include a CT scan of the chest and abdomen, PET scan, with the addition of EUS for patients with apparent locoregional disease.

Complete Resection

The importance of an R0 resection has been demonstrated time and again in numerous malig-nancies, and multiple studies have specifically demonstrated a survival benefit of an R0 resection in esophageal cancer. A summary of selected studies supporting the importance of negative margins can be seen in **Table 10**.

A large propensity score matched study by Markar and colleagues[46] demonstrated that a microscopically positive margin was an indepen-dent predictor of poor prognosis for patients un-dergoing esophagectomy. They retrospectively analyzed survival from a group of more than 2800 subjects and found that an R1 resection increased the HR of both mortality and recurrence. Survival was decreased substantially for both sub-jects with node-positive disease (66.0 vs 24.4 months) and node-negative disease (23.0 vs 16.6 months). Another, smaller, single-center study by Wang and colleagues[47] examined the impact of a positive proximal resection margin on survival, also through propensity score matching, and demonstrated a similar survival benefit of R0 resection (68.0 vs 25.0 months). These investiga-tors also found improved survival with adjuvant therapy in subjects with R1 resection, although this remains controversial.

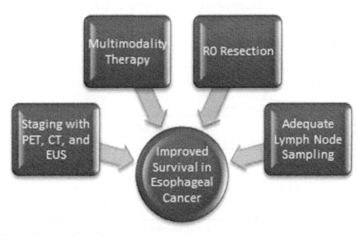

Fig. 4. Quality indicators in esophageal cancer.

Table 9
A summary of studies supporting staging with PET, computed tomography, and endoscopic ultrasound for esophageal cancer

Study	Design Year of Study	Number of Subjects	Conclusions
PET			
Systematic review of the staging performance of 18F-fluorodeoxyglucose positron emission tomography in esophageal cancer[41]	Systematic review (2004)	12 studies n = 421 for nodal analysis n = 452 for metastatic analysis	PET is helpful for detecting regional and distant metastases • Sensitivity and specificity were as follows: ○ Nodal: 51%, 84% ○ Distant: 67%, 97%
EUS			
Staging accuracy of esophageal cancer by EUS[42]	Meta-analysis and systematic review (2008)	49 studies n = 2558	EUS is sensitive and specific for tumor and node staging • EUS is more accurate in higher than lower stage disease • EUS performs better than PET and CT in identifying mediastinal disease • Sensitivity and specificity by stage were as follows: ○ T1: 82%, 99% ○ T2: 81%, 96% ○ T3: 91%, 94% ○ T4: 92%, 97% ○ N: 85%, 85%
Comparison of EUS, PET, and CT			
Staging investigations for esophageal cancer[43]	Meta-analysis (2008)		EUS is the most sensitive for detecting lymph node metastases, but CT and PET are more specific Sensitivity and specificity by modality were as follows: • EUS ○ N: 80%, 70% • CT ○ N: 50%, 83% ○ M: 52%, 91% • PET ○ N: 57%, 85% ○ M: 71%, 93%

Data from Refs.[41–43]

Rüdiger Siewert and colleagues[51] conducted a large cohort study of more than 1000 subjects that also demonstrated that R0 resection was a dominant factor in multivariate analysis that significantly predicted overall survival for esophageal subjects with cancer both at 5 years (38.7% vs 13.7%) and at 10 years (28.3% vs 11.6%). Another 10-year single-center series of more than 200 subjects by Mulligan and colleagues[48] demonstrated decreased tumor recurrence and a significant increase in survival with an R0 resection.

Adequate Lymphadenectomy

Numerous studies have shown a survival benefit in esophageal cancer with increasing extent of lymphadenectomy. A summary of relevant primary studies with recommended LN counts can be seen in **Table 11**.

Table 10
A summary of studies supporting the importance of an R0 resection for esophageal cancer

Study	Design Year of Study	Number of Subjects	Conclusions
Significance of microscopically incomplete resection margin after esophagectomy for esophageal cancer[46]	Multicenter retrospective study: propensity score matched 1:3 (2016)	2815	R1 resection margin was an independent predictor of poor prognosis • Increased mortality with a HR of 1.57 • Increased recurrence with a HR of 1.56 • Survival with N0 disease was 66.0 mo with R0 resection vs 24.4 mo with R1 resection • Survival with N1 disease was 23.0 mo with R0 resection vs 16.6 mo with R1 resection
Positive esophageal proximal resection margin: an important prognostic factor for esophageal cancer that warrants adjuvant therapy[47]	Single-center retrospective study: propensity score matched 1:2 (2016)	111	R1 proximal resection margin conveyed worse prognosis • Survival was 68.0 mo with R0 resection vs 35.0 mo with R1 resection
Margin involvement and outcome in esophageal carcinoma: a 10-y experience in a specialist unit[48]	Single-center cohort (2004)	212	Negative margins were associated with decreased cancer recurrence and improved survival (RR 2.16) on multivariate analysis
Extent of esophageal resection for adenocarcinoma of the esophagogastric junction[49]	Retrospective cohort (2003)	94	Positive margins affected survival • Survival was 36.3 mo with R0 resection vs 11.1 mo with R1 resection
Surgical therapy for adenocarcinoma of the cardia: modalities of recurrence and extension of resection[50]	Retrospective cohort (2001)	116	Survival was correlated with microscopically positive margins • Survival was 31.0 mo with R0 resection vs 18.0 mo with R1 resection
Adenocarcinoma of the esophagogastric junction: Results of surgical therapy based on anatomic or topographic classifications in 1002 consecutive subjects[51]	Single-center cohort (2000)	1002	R0 resection was among the most important prognostic factors on multivariate analysis • 5-y survival was 38.7% with R0 resection vs 13.7% with R1/R2 resection • 10-y survival was 28.3% with R0 resection vs 11.6% with R1/R2 resection

Data from Refs.[46–51]

Table 11
A summary of studies supporting increased extent of lymphadenectomy

Study	Design Year of Study	Number of Subjects	Recommendations
WECC guidelines for lymphadenectomy predict survival following neoadjuvant therapy[52]	Prospective cohort (2012)	135	>10 for T1 or less >20 for T2 >30 for T3/4
Optimum lymphadenectomy for esophageal cancer[53]	Retrospective review from WECC database (2010)	4627	For N0 cancers: • 10–12 for pT1 • 15–22 for pT2 • 31–42 for pT3/4 For N1-2 cancers: • 10 for pT1 • 15 for pT2 • 29–50 for pT3/4
Total number of lymph nodes predicts survival in esophageal cancer[54]	Retrospective review of single-institution database (2008)	264	Overall survival improved with increasing lymphadenectomy
The number of lymph nodes removed predicts survival in esophageal cancer: an international study on the impact of extent of surgical resection[55]	Retrospective database review, data compiled from 9 international centers (2008)	2303	>23 lymph nodes
Effects of the number of lymph nodes sampled on postoperative survival of lymph node-negative esophageal cancer[56]	Retrospective database review based on SEER (2008)	972	>18 lymph nodes
Clinical impact of lymphadenectomy extent in resectable esophageal cancer[57]	Retrospective database review based on SEER (2007)	2597	>30 lymph nodes >15 negative lymph nodes
The prognostic importance of the number of involved lymph nodes in esophageal cancer: implications for revision of the AJCC staging system[58]	Retrospective review, single-institution (2006)	336	>18 lymph nodes for diagnostic accuracy
Staging of esophageal carcinoma: length of tumor and number of involved regional lymph nodes. Are these independent prognostic factors?[59]	Single-institution study (2006)	213	>15 negative lymph nodes

Data from Refs.[52–59]

A study[53] based on Worldwide Esophageal Cancer Collaboration (WECC) database of more than 4500 subjects explored the number of LNs that should be examined by stage of disease in subjects undergoing upfront surgery. They found that for any pathologic node-negative cancers that were moderately or poorly differentiated, as well as for all cancers with positive nodes, a more extensive lymphadenectomy was associated with improved 5-year survival. Additionally, they suggested the following minimum LN counts were optimal based on pathologic tumor (pT) status: 10 nodes for pT1, 20 nodes for pT2, and 30 nodes for pT3 or greater. Stiles and colleagues[52] aimed to apply these guidelines to 135 subjects who had received neoadjuvant treatment and found that having a guideline-supported lymphadenectomy was predictive of survival, but this was also highly correlated with postinduction pathologic tumor staging.

Peyre and colleagues[55] conducted a multicenter database study of more than 2000 subjects to identify a threshold for benefit of LN removal and found that 23 nodes were optimal. Similar to what was observed in the WECC study, they noted

the benefit of this more extensive lymphadenectomy was greater for higher stage disease.

A pair of studies examined the impact of the extent of lymphadenectomy using Surveillance, Epidemiology, and End Results (SEER) data. Schwarz and colleagues[57] examined more than 2500 subjects and quantified the relative increase in overall survival per 10 additional LNs resected and found it increased 4% to 5%. They found that both negative LN counts greater than 15 and total LN counts greater than 30 were associated

Table 12
A summary of studies supporting induction chemoradiation for locally advanced esophageal cancer

Study	Design, Year of Study	Number of Subjects	Conclusions
Preoperative chemoradiotherapy for esophageal or junctional cancer (CROSS)[60,61]	Randomized controlled trial (2012)	366	Favored induction chemoradiation • T1N1, T2-3N0-1 subjects • No difference in perioperative mortality or complication rates • Survival was 49.4 mo with CRT vs 24.0 mo with surgery alone
Neoadjuvant chemoradiotherapy plus surgery vs surgery alone for esophageal or junctional cancer (CROSS): long-term results of a randomized controlled trial[62]	Randomized controlled trial, long-term follow-up for initial CROSS trial (2015)	366	Favored induction chemoradiation • T1N1, T2-3N0-1 subjects • Confirmed findings from the initial CROSS trial remained true long-term • Adenocarcinoma survival: 43.2 mo with CRT vs 27.1 mo with surgery alone • Squamous cell carcinoma survival: 81.6 mo with CRT vs 21.1 mo with surgery alone
Phase III trial of trimodality therapy with cisplatin, fluorouracil, radiotherapy, and surgery compared with surgery alone for esophageal cancer: CALGB 9781[63]	Randomized controlled trial (2008)	56	Favored induction chemoradiation • T2-3N0-1, T4N0 subjects • No difference in treatment mortality or postoperative complication rates • Survival was 4.48 y with CRT vs 1.79 y with surgery alone
A comparison of multimodal therapy and surgery for esophageal adenocarcinoma[64]	Randomized controlled trial (1996)	102	Favored induction chemoradiation • Survival was 16 mo with CRT vs 11 mo with surgery alone based on intention to treat • Survival was 32 mo with CRT vs 11 mo with surgery alone based on treatment received

Abbreviations: CALGB, cancer and leukemia group B; CROSS, chemoradiotherapy for oesophageal cancer followed by surgery study; CRT, chemoradiotherapy.
  Data from Refs.[60–64]

with improved overall survival. These findings were consistent with additional single-institution studies.[54,59] Using the SEER data, Greenstein and colleagues[56] confirmed that increasing LN count was associated with improved survival but settled on 18 as the optimal number, consistent with the number Rizk and colleagues[58] had identified as needed for accurate staging through recursive partitioning analysis of an institutional database of more than 300 subjects.

The data overall are clear that a more extensive lymphadenectomy improves the accuracy of staging and observed overall survival, though it remains debatable how much of the observed survival benefit is due to stage migration. NCCN guidelines[45] recommend that at least 15 LNs are removed and pathologically examined across all stages of esophageal cancer, though evidence from the primary literature is clearly mixed with regard to the optimal count, especially following induction chemoradiation.

Induction Chemoradiation

Randomized controlled trials have shown a survival benefit of induction chemoradiation for stage IIB or higher esophageal cancer. A summary of these studies can be seen in **Table 12**.

The primary trial supporting induction therapy for locally advanced esophageal cancer was the CROSS trial (Chemoradiotherapy for Oesophageal cancer followed by Surgery Study).[60,61] This randomized controlled trial included more than 350 subjects with esophageal cancer, 75% of which had adenocarcinoma, who were clinically staged as T1N1, T2-3N0-1. This trial randomized subjects to induction chemoradiation versus surgery and found no difference in perioperative mortality or morbidity with a substantial increase in overall median survival for the induction therapy group (49.4 vs 24.0 months), as well as a decrease in ultimate esophageal cancer specific mortality (85% vs 94%), with very low rates of chemoradiation mortality (0.6%) and failure to proceed to surgery (6.0%). When these subjects did undergo resection, they also were much more likely to get an R0 resection (92% vs 69%). A 5-year follow-up study of the CROSS subjects[62] revealed that the initially observed survival benefits persisted, and provided data on the median survival benefit difference between squamous cell and adenocarcinoma.

This landmark trial was preceded by 2 other older randomized trials that showed a benefit of induction chemoradiation. The CALGB 9781 trial (Cancer and Leukemia Group B)[63] enrolled more than 50 subjects and also randomized subjects

to preoperative chemoradiation or surgery alone and demonstrated a survival benefit (4.48 vs 1.79 years), no difference in complications (24 reported complications in each group), and no difference in mortality (1 infection-related mortality in the induction group and 1 perioperative death in the surgery group). Similarly, Walsh and colleagues[64] enrolled more than 100 subjects who were randomized to induction therapy versus surgery alone. Again, there was a demonstrated benefit for trimodality therapy.

STS practice guidelines[65] are supported by this evidence and include that patients with locally advanced disease should undergo preoperative chemoradiation, should be restaged following induction therapy, and should undergo surgical resection even in the setting of complete pathologic response. The NCCN guidelines[45] also support preoperative chemoradiation followed by an assessment of response.

SUMMARY

In conclusion, there is substantial evidence that quality metrics within process and outcome measures can be identified for lung and esophageal cancer, and that adhering to evidence-based quality recommendations have implications for survival in thoracic malignancies. Furthermore, prior studies show that adherence to these metrics remains suboptimal. We must continue to strive toward further refining these measures and achieving greater adherence to established ones.

REFERENCES

1. Donabedian A. Evaluating the quality of medical care. Milbank Mem Fund Q 1966;33(4):691–729.
2. Darling G, Malthaner R, Dickie J, et al. Quality indicators for non-small cell lung cancer operations with use of a modified Delphi consensus process. Ann Thorac Surg 2014;98(1):183–90.
3. Numan RC, Berge MT, Burgers JA, et al. Peri- and postoperative management of stage I–III Non Small Cell Lung Cancer: Which quality of care indicators are evidence-based? Lung Cancer 2016;101:129–36.
4. Numan RC, Berge MT, Burgers JA, et al. Pre- and postoperative care for stage I–III NSCLC: Which quality of care indicators are evidence-based? Lung Cancer 2016;101:120–8.
5. Rivera MP, Mehta AC, Wahidi MM. Establishing the diagnosis of lung cancer. Chest 2013;143(5): e142S–165.
6. Samson P, Patel A, Garrett T, et al. Effects of delayed surgical resection on short-term and long-term outcomes in clinical stage i non-small cell lung cancer. Ann Thorac Surg 2015;99(6):1906–13.

7. NCCN Clinical Practice Guidelines in Oncology: Non-Small Cell Lung Cancer (National Comprehensive Cancer Network). 2017. Available at: https://www.nccn.org/professionals/physician_gls/pdf/nscl.pdf. Accessed March 29, 2017.

8. British Thoracic Society, Society of Cardiothoracic Surgeons of Great Britain and Ireland Working Party. BTS guidelines: guidelines on the selection of patients with lung cancer for surgery. Thorax 2001; 56(2):89–108. Available at: http://www.ncbi.nlm.nih.gov/pubmed/11209097. Accessed March 29, 2017.

9. Howington JA, Blum MG, Chang AC, et al. Treatment of stage I and II non-small cell lung cancer: Diagnosis and management of lung cancer, 3rd ed: American college of chest physicians evidence-based clinical practice guidelines. Chest 2013; 143(5 Suppl):e314S–340.

10. Detterbeck FC, Lewis SZ, Diekemper R, et al. Executive summary: diagnosis and management of lung cancer, 3rd ed: American College of Chest Physicians evidence-based clinical practice guidelines. Chest 2013;143(5):7S–37S.

11. Ramnath N, Dilling TJ, Harris LJ, et al. Treatment of stage III non-small cell lung cancer. Chest 2013; 143(5):e314S–340.

12. Surgeons TS of T, ed. General Thoracic Surgery Database Data Collection. STS National Database Data Managers. 2016. Available at: http://www.sts.org/quality-research-patient-safety/national-database/database-managers/general-thoracic-surgery-databa-1. Accessed March 29, 2017.

13. Little AG, Rusch VW, Bonner JA, et al. Patterns of surgical care of lung cancer patients. Ann Thorac Surg 2005;80(6):2051–6 [discussion: 2056].

14. Silvestri GA, Gonzalez AV, Jantz MA, et al. Methods for staging non-small cell lung cancer. Chest 2013; 143(5):e211S–250.

15. Detterbeck FC, Jantz MA, Wallace M, et al. Invasive mediastinal staging of lung cancer: ACCP evidence-based clinical practice guidelines (2nd edition). Chest 2007;132(3 Suppl):202s–20s.

16. Lardinoise D, Weder W, Hany TF, et al. Staging of non–small-cell lung cancer with Integrated Positron-Emission Tomography and Computed Tomography. N Engl J Med 2003;348(25):2500–7.

17. Pieterman RM, van Putten JWG, Meuzelaar JJ, et al. Preoperative staging of non–small-cell lung cancer with Positron-Emission Tomography. N Engl J Med 2000;343(4):254–61.

18. Farjah F, Flum DR, Ramsey SD, et al. Multi-modality mediastinal staging for lung cancer among medicare beneficiaries. J Thorac Oncol 2009;4(3):355–63.

19. Herder GJM, Kramer H, Hoekstra OS, et al. Traditional versus up-front [18F] fluorodeoxyglucose-positron emission tomography staging of non-small-cell lung cancer: A Dutch cooperative randomized study. J Clin Oncol 2006;24(12):1800–6.

20. Viney RC, Boyer MJ, King MT, et al. Randomized controlled trial of the role of positron emission tomography in the management of stage I and II non-small-cell lung cancer. J Clin Oncol 2004; 22(12):2357–62.

21. Labarca G, Aravena C, Ortega F, et al. Minimally invasive methods for staging in lung cancer: systematic review and meta-analysis. Pulm Med 2016; 2016:1024709.

22. National Lung Screening Trial Research Team, Aberle DR, Adams AM, et al. Reduced lung-cancer mortality with low-dose Computed Tomographic Screening. N Engl J Med 2011;365(5): 395–409.

23. Bilimoria KY, Ko CY, Tomlinson JS, et al. Wait times for cancer surgery in the United States: trends and predictors of delays. Ann Surg 2011;253(4):779–85.

24. Lathan CS, Neville BA, Earle CC. The effect of race on invasive staging and surgery in non-small-cell lung cancer. J Clin Oncol 2006;24(3):413–8.

25. Yorio JT, Yan J, Xie Y, et al. Socioeconomic disparities in lung cancer treatment and outcomes persist within a single academic medical center. Clin Lung Cancer 2012;13(6):448–57.

26. Lung Measure Specifications Cancer Programs Practice Profile Reports (CP 3 R). Available at: https://www.facs.org/~/media/files/quality%20programs/cancer/ncdb/measure%20specs%20nscl.ashx. Accessed March 29, 2017.

27. Brunelli A, Charloux A, Bolliger CT, et al. ERS/ESTS clinical guidelines on fitness for radical therapy in lung cancer patients (surgery and chemo-radiotherapy). Eur Respir J 2009;34(1):17–41.

28. Colice GL, Shafazand S, Griffin JP, et al. Physiologic evaluation of the patient with lung cancer being considered for resectional surgery: ACCP evidenced-based clinical practice guidelines (2nd edition). Chest 2007; 132(3 Suppl.):161s–77s.

29. Yang H-X, Woo KM, Sima CS, et al. Long-term survival based on the surgical approach to lobectomy for clinical stage I nonsmall cell lung cancer: comparison of robotic, video-assisted thoracic surgery, and thoracotomy lobectomy. Ann Surg 2017; 265(2):431–7.

30. Gajra A, Newman N, Gamble GP, et al. Effect of number of lymph nodes sampled on outcome in patients with stage I non-small-cell lung cancer. J Clin Oncol 2003;21(6):1029–34.

31. Keller SM, Adak S, Wagner H, et al. Mediastinal lymph node dissection improves survival in patients with stages II and IIIa non-small cell lung cancer. Ann Thorac Surg 2000;70(2):358–65.

32. Samson P, Crabtree T, Broderick S, et al. Quality measures in clinical stage I non-small cell lung cancer: improved performance is associated with improved survival. Ann Thorac Surg 2017;103(1): 303–11.

33. The Society of Thoracic Surgeons. Quality Performance Measures | STS. 2017. Available at: http://www.sts.org/quality-research-patient-safety/quality/quality-performance-measures. Accessed March 29, 2017.

34. Burdett S, Rydzewska L, Tierney J, et al. Postoperative radiotherapy for non-small cell lung cancer. Cochrane Database Syst Rev 2016;(10):CD002142.

35. Riquet M, Achour K, Foucault C, et al. Microscopic residual disease after resection for lung cancer: a multifaceted but poor factor of prognosis. Ann Thorac Surg 2010;89(3):870–5.

36. Wind J, Smit EJ, Senan S, et al. Residual disease at the bronchial stump after curative resection for lung cancer. Eur J Cardiothorac Surg 2007;32(1):29–34.

37. Evans W, Ung Y, Assouad N. Improving the quality of lung cancer care in ontario: the lung cancer disease pathway initiative. J Thorac Oncol 2013;8(7):876–82.

38. Courrech Staal EFW, Wouters MWJM, Boot H, et al. Quality-of-care indicators for oesophageal cancer surgery: A review. Eur J Surg Oncol 2010;36(11):1035–43.

39. Samson P, Puri V, Broderick S, et al. Adhering to quality measures in esophagectomy is associated with improved survival in all stages of esophageal cancer. Ann Thorac Surg 2017;103:1101–8.

40. Molena D, Mungo B, Stem M, et al. Does quality of care matter? A study of adherence to national comprehensive cancer network guidelines for patients with locally advanced esophageal cancer. J Gastrointest Surg 2015;19(10):1739–47.

41. van Westreenen HL, Westerterp M, Bossuyt PMM, et al. Systematic review of the staging performance of 18F-fluorodeoxyglucose Positron Emission Tomography in esophageal cancer. J Clin Oncol 2004;22(18):3805–12.

42. Puli SR, Reddy JBK, Bechtold ML, et al. Staging accuracy of esophageal cancer by endoscopic ultrasound: A meta-analysis and systematic review. World J Gastroenterol 2008;14(10):1479–90.

43. van Vliet EPM, Heijenbrok-Kal MH, Hunink MGM, et al. Staging investigations for oesophageal cancer: a meta-analysis. Br J Cancer 2008;98(3):547–57.

44. Varghese TK, Hofstetter WL, Rizk NP, et al. The society of thoracic surgeons guidelines on the diagnosis and staging of patients with esophageal cancer. Ann Thorac Surg 2013;96(1):346–56.

45. Nicole McMillian N, Hema Sundar M, Gibson M, et al. MPH Dana-Farber/Brigham and Women's Cancer Center NCCN Guidelines Version 2.2016 updates esophageal and esophagogastric junction cancers. Available at: https://www.nccn.org/professionals/physician_gls/pdf/esophageal.pdf. Accessed March 2, 2017.

46. Markar SR, Gronnier C, Duhamel A, et al. Significance of microscopically incomplete resection margin after esophagectomy for esophageal cancer. Ann Surg 2016;263(4):712–8.

47. Wang Y-C, Deng H-Y, Wang W-P, et al. Positive esophageal proximal resection margin: an important prognostic factor for esophageal cancer that warrants adjuvant therapy. J Thorac Dis 2016;8(9):2512–8.

48. Mulligan ED, Dunne B, Griffin M, et al. Margin involvement and outcome in oesophageal carcinoma: A 10-year experience in a specialist unit. Eur J Surg Oncol 2004;30(3):313–7.

49. Mariette C, Castel B, Balon JM, et al. Extent of oesophageal resection for adenocarcinoma of the oesophagogastric junction. Eur J Surg Oncol 2003;29(7):588–93.

50. Mattioli S, Di Simone MP, Ferruzzi L, et al. Surgical therapy for adenocarcinoma of the cardia: Modalities of recurrence and extension of resection. Dis Esophagus 2001;14(2):104–9.

51. Rüdiger Siewert J, Feith M, Werner M, et al. Adenocarcinoma of the esophagogastric junction: results of surgical therapy based on anatomical/topographic classification in 1,002 consecutive patients. Ann Surg 2000;232(3):353–61.

52. Stiles BM, Nasar A, Mirza FA, et al. Worldwide oesophageal cancer collaboration guidelines for lymphadenectomy predict survival following neoadjuvant therapy. Eur J Cardiothorac Surg 2012;42(4):659–64.

53. Rizk NP, Ishwaran H, Rice TW, et al. Optimum lymphadenectomy for esophageal cancer. Ann Surg 2010;251(1):46–50.

54. Altorki NK, Zhou XK, Stiles B, et al. Total number of resected lymph nodes predicts survival in esophageal cancer. Ann Surg 2008;248(2):221–6.

55. Peyre CG, Hagen JA, DeMeester SR, et al. The number of lymph nodes removed predicts survival in esophageal cancer: an international study on the impact of extent of surgical resection. Ann Surg 2008;248(4):549–56.

56. Greenstein AJ, Litle VR, Swanson SJ, et al. Effect of the number of lymph nodes sampled on postoperative survival of lymph node-negative esophageal cancer. Cancer 2008;112(6):1239–46.

57. Schwarz RE, Smith DD. Clinical impact of lymphadenectomy extent in resectable esophageal cancer. J Gastrointest Surg 2007;11(11):1384–94.

58. Rizk N, Venkatraman E, Park B, et al. The prognostic importance of the number of involved lymph nodes in esophageal cancer: Implications for revisions of the American Joint Committee on Cancer staging system. J Thorac Cardiovasc Surg 2006;132(6):1374–81.e2.

59. Bollschweiler E, Baldus SE, Schröder W, et al. Staging of esophageal carcinoma: Length of tumor and number of involved regional lymph nodes. Are these independent prognostic factors? J Surg Oncol 2006;94(5):355–63.

60. van Hagen P, Hulshof MCCM, van Lanschot JJB, et al. Preoperative chemoradiotherapy for esophageal or junctional cancer. N Engl J Med 2012; 366(22):2074–84.

61. van Heijl M, van Lanschot JJB, Koppert LB, et al. Neoadjuvant chemoradiation followed by surgery versus surgery alone for patients with adenocarcinoma or squamous cell carcinoma of the esophagus (CROSS). BMC Surg 2008;8(1):21.

62. Shapiro J, van Lanschot JJB, Hulshof MCCM, et al. Neoadjuvant chemoradiotherapy plus surgery versus surgery alone for oesophageal or junctional cancer (CROSS): Long-term results of a randomised controlled trial. Lancet Oncol 2015;16(9):1090–8.

63. Tepper J, Krasna MJ, Niedzwiecki D, et al. Phase III trial of trimodality therapy with cisplatin, fluorouracil, radiotherapy, and surgery compared with surgery alone for esophageal cancer: CALGB 9781. J Clin Oncol 2008;26(7):1086–92.

64. Walsh TN, Noonan N, Hollywood D, et al. A Comparison of Multimodal Therapy and Surgery for Esophageal Adenocarcinoma. N Engl J Med 1996;335(7):462–7.

65. Little AG, Lerut AE, Harpole DH, et al. The Society of Thoracic Surgeons practice guidelines on the role of multimodality treatment for cancer of the esophagus and gastroesophageal junction. Ann Thorac Surg 2014;98(5):1880–5.

66. Reifel JL, Asch SM, Kerr EA, et al. Quality of care for oncologic conditions and HIV: a review of the literature and quality indicators. Arlington (VA): RAND Corporation; 2000.

National Quality Forum Metrics for Thoracic Surgery

Anthony Cipriano, MD, William R. Burfeind Jr, MD*

KEYWORDS

- National Quality Forum • Lung cancer • Esophageal cancer • Endorsed measures

KEY POINTS

- The NQF is a multistakeholder, nonprofit, membership-based organization that tries to improve health care through the preferential use of valid performance measures.
- The NQF uses a multistep, formal, consensus development process to evaluate and endorse potential measures that are created by either public or private groups.
- The Society of Thoracic Surgeons has the most endorsed measures, 34, of any specialty medical society. These include six endorsed general thoracic surgery measures, four pediatric cardiac surgery measures, and 24 adult cardiac surgery measures.
- The endorsed general thoracic surgery measures include one structure measure, two process measures, and three risk-adjusted models of morbidity and mortality after lung and esophageal resection. They represent the only NQF-endorsed measures for general thoracic surgery.

INTRODUCTION

Measuring surgeon performance has become an essential professional responsibility for surgeons.[1] Professional societies have incorporated performance measurement and quality improvement into their maintenance of certification.[2,3] Not only does performance improvement help define quality but it is increasingly linked directly to payment through value-based purchasing and accountable care arrangements.[4] It is likely that most surgeons reading this article have some of their salary directly tied to quality-based incentive compensation plans. The Society of Thoracic Surgeons (STS) has been at the leading edge of surgeon performance measurement, analysis, and patient safety through the three national databases: (1) Adult Cardiac Surgery Database, (2) General Thoracic Surgery Database, and (3) Congenital Heart Surgery Database.[5] The STS commitment to performance improvement is also evidenced by the fact that they have developed 34 quality measures that have been endorsed by the National Quality Forum (NQF) (**Table 1**). The NQF is the federally designated organization responsible for recommending measures for use in payment and public reporting programs.[6]

WHAT IS THE NATIONAL QUALITY FORUM?

NQF is a private, nonprofit, membership-based organization that promotes the continual improvement of national health care quality by means of using reliable quality measures and public reporting. It is the only consensus-based health care organization in the nation, as defined by the Office of Management and Budget, and as such, the federal government relies on the consensus-standards endorsed by the NQF to measure and publically report on performance in the health care setting.[6]

Disclosure: Neither author has any commercial or financial conflicts of interest related to this article.
Department of Surgery, St. Luke's University Health Network, 701 Ostrum Street, Suite 603, Bethlehem, PA 18015, USA
* Corresponding author.
E-mail address: william.burfeind@sluhn.org

Thorac Surg Clin 27 (2017) 245–249
http://dx.doi.org/10.1016/j.thorsurg.2017.03.003

Table 1
NQF endorsed measures sponsored by the STS

NQF No.	General Thoracic Surgery Measures
Cip0455	Recording of clinical stage before surgery for lung or esophageal cancer resection
0456	Participation in a systematic national database for general thoracic surgery
0457	Recording of performance status before lung or esophageal cancer resection
0459	Risk-adjusted morbidity: length of stay >14 days after elective lobectomy for lung cancer
0460	Risk-adjusted morbidity and mortality for esophagectomy for cancer
1790	Risk-adjusted morbidity and mortality for lung resection for lung cancer

NQF No.	Adult Cardiac Surgery Measures
0113	Participation in a systematic database for cardiac surgery
0114	Risk-adjusted postoperative renal failure
0115	Risk-adjusted surgical re-exploration
0116	Antiplatelet medication on discharge
0117	β-Blockade on discharge
0118	Antilipid treatment on discharge
0119	Risk-adjusted operative mortality for CABG
0120	Risk-adjusted operative mortality for aortic valve replacement
0121	Risk-adjusted operative mortality for mitral valve replacement
0122	Risk-adjusted operative mortality for mitral valve replacement + CABG
0123	Risk-adjusted operative mortality for aortic valve replacement + CABG
0126	Selection of antibiotic prophylaxis for cardiac surgery patients
0127	Preoperative β-blockade
0128	Duration of antibiotic prophylaxis in cardiac surgery patients
0129	Risk-adjusted postoperative prolonged intubation (ventilation)
0130	Risk-adjusted deep sternal wound infection
0131	Risk-adjusted stroke/cerebrovascular accident
0134	Use of internal mammary artery in CAGB
0696	STS CABG composite score
1501	Risk-adjusted operative mortality for mitral valve repair
1502	Risk-adjusted operative mortality for mitral valve repair + CABG
2514	Risk-adjusted CABG readmission rate
2561	STS aortic valve replacement composite score
2563	STS aortic valve replacement + CABG composite score

NQF No.	Pediatric Cardiac Surgery Measures
0732	Surgical volume for pediatric and congenital heart surgery: total programmatic volume and programmatic volume stratified by the five STS-EACTS mortality categories
0733	Operative mortality stratified by the five STAT mortality categories
0734	Participation in a national database for pediatric and congenital heart surgery
2683	Risk-adjusted operative mortality for pediatric and congenital heart surgery

Abbreviations: CABG, coronary artery bypass graft; STAT, Society of Thoracic Surgeons - European Association of Thoracic Surgery.
Data from https://www.qualityforum.org/. Accessed October 1, 2016.

As of 2016, the NQF recognizes more than 400 members including public and private health agencies, health care provider organizations, consumer groups, health care purchasers, and research and quality improvement organizations.[7]

BRIEF HISTORY OF THE NATIONAL QUALITY FORUM

Demands for greater health care accountability culminated in the release of three independently conducted reviews published in 1998. Reports by RAND, another by the Institute of Medicine's National Roundtable on Health Care Quality, and the third by the President's Advisory Commission on Consumer Protection and Quality in the Health Care Industry clearly recognized health care errors as a serious public health problem.[8–10] The President's Advisory Commission therefore proposed a dual public/private partnership between two organizations: the private National Forum on Health Care Quality Measurement and Reporting and the public, Advisory Council for Health Care Quality.[11] The Advisory Council was to identify and set national goals for health care quality improvement, whereas the Quality Forum was to devise ways to standardize the measurement of health care quality and reporting with the ultimate aim of advancing the goals set forth by the Advisory Council. The NQF was launched in 1999; however, the Advisory Council, to date, has not been established.

WHY IS THE NATIONAL QUALITY FORUM IMPORTANT?

NQF-endorsed measures are considered the gold standard for health care measurement in the United States.[6] Not only do these consensus-measures define how provider performance is compared and tracked against national benchmarks, but they also serve as the measures that dictate performance-based reimbursement. Currently, about 300 NQF-endorsed measures are used in more than 20 federal, public reporting, and pay-for-performance programs.[6]

How Does a Measure Get Endorsed?

The NQF uses a multistep, formal, consensus development process to evaluate and endorse potential measures that are created by either public or private groups. Before a proposed measure is even considered for endorsement, it must meet six conditions, two of which are that the measure has been tested for reliability and validity, and the intended use of the measure includes accountability or public reporting applications and performance improvement.[6] If all conditions for consideration are met, the proposed measure then is evaluated against five criteria in the following order: (1) importance to measure and report, (2) scientific acceptability of measure properties, (3) feasibility, (4) usability, and (5) related and competing measures.

Previously endorsed measures are re-evaluated against the same criteria approximately every 3 years. Currently, the NQF endorses approximately 630 measures that include process measures, cost measures, efficiency measures, outcome measures, and structure measures.

GENERAL THORACIC MEASURES

In 2007, the STS submitted six general thoracic measures for consideration of endorsement by the NQF. The measures included one structure measure: participating in a national database for general thoracic surgery (0456). Three process measures are (1) recording of performance status before resection for lung or esophagus cancer (0457) (2) recording of clinical stage before lung and esophageal resection (0455) and (3) performing lung function tests before major anatomic pulmonary resection (0458). There were also two outcome measures: "risk-adjusted morbidity after lobectomy for lung cancer" (0459) and "risk-adjusted mortality after esophagectomy for esophagus cancer" (0460). In early 2008 all the measures were endorsed.

In 2010, all the STS general thoracic measures were re-endorsed. Additionally, at this time, two articles had been published that directly supported the two endorsed outcomes measures. The first, in 2008, was Wright and colleagues[12] article, which examined the first 4979 lobectomies within the database and confirmed that mortality was low at 1.4% and individual complications were rare. Prolonged length of stay (PLOS) greater than 14 days was modeled as a surrogate marker for postoperative complications and was shown to be statistically valid. PLOS happened in 7% of the patients and those patients had higher discharge mortality (10.8% vs 0.7%). Predictors of PLOS included advancing age, Zubrod score, American Society of Anesthesiologists (ASA) score, male gender, insulin-dependent diabetes, renal dysfunction, induction therapy, and smoking status. Video-assisted approach was protective. The second article supporting an outcome measure, also from Wright and coworkers,[13] examined the first 2315 esophagectomies in the database and a risk model was generated that allowed individual STS sites to compare their results with those of the other STS sites. The overall analysis demonstrated a low operative mortality of 2.7%. Predictors of morbidity and mortality included advancing age or ASA score, congestive heart failure, coronary heart disease, peripheral vascular disease, hypertension, insulin-dependent diabetes, and cigarette smoking. The analysis failed to show a strong volume performance relationship for the composite measure among STS General Thoracic Surgery Database participants. An important limitation to the volume analysis was that for the model to be statistically valid, programs performing fewer than six esophagectomies in 6 years (29/73 programs; 40%) were excluded. Despite this limitation, the composite of morbidity and mortality for programs performing one esophagectomy per year did not look different from programs with much higher volumes.

In the 2012 cycle, all the currently endorsed measures were re-endorsed. A new outcome measure entitled "risk-adjusted morbidity and mortality for lung resection for lung cancer" (1790) was endorsed, bringing the total STS general thoracic surgery measures to seven. With the endorsement of this measure, the previously endorsed measure, 0459, had its name changed to "risk-adjusted morbidity: prolonged length of stay greater than 14 days after elective lobectomy for lung cancer." The new measure, 1790, was based on the model run for the STS database participant's biannual report and published by Kozower and coworkers.[14] By 2010, there were enough lung cancer resections in the database to model morbidity and mortality separately rather than relying on PLOS as a surrogate for complications. There were three models generated examining the risk-adjusted outcomes of mortality, major morbidity, and the composite of mortality or major morbidity. More than 18,000 patients who had had lobectomy, bilobectomy, segmentectomy, pneumonectomy, or wedge resection for lung cancer were included in the models. The STS General Thoracic Surgery Database participants were demonstrated to have a perioperative mortality of 2.2%, a major morbidity rate of 7.9%, and composite morbidity and mortality of 8.6% for lung cancer resections. In addition to the risk models, this article described an analysis of hospital performance variation. Performance variation was summarized by calculating hospital-specific standardized incidence ratios or the ratio of a participating hospitals risk-adjusted rate divided by the risk-adjusted rate of a hypothetical average STS participant. By applying Bayesian 95% probability intervals, centers with better or worse than expected performance could be distinguished.

In 2014, the NQF measure evaluation form stated that developers must clearly demonstrate that a process measure has a direct impact on or link to a desired health outcome in the target population. As such, the process measure of obtaining pulmonary function tests before anatomic pulmonary resection was voluntarily removed.

For the 2016 cycle, the STS general thoracic surgery measures were transitioned out of the surgery standing committee for the NQF and into the cancer standing committee. The STS plans to withdraw two more process measures, "recording of performance status before lung and esophageal resection" (0457) and "recording of clinical stage before surgery for lung cancer and esophageal cancer resection" (0455). Two outcome measures, "risk-adjusted morbidity: length of stay greater than 14 days after elective lobectomy for lung cancer" (0459) and "risk-adjusted morbidity and mortality for esophagectomy for cancer" (0460) are being re-evaluated and may not be endorsed. The need for measure 0459, which uses a surrogate marker, PLOS, to examine morbidity, has been questioned because the STS has a risk-adjusted measure that directly addresses morbidity and mortality for lung cancer resection (1790). For measure 0460, the cancer standing committee is currently debating about the reliability of the measure. Of specific concern was that the reliability of the model decreased with decreasing numbers of cases performed at each site and that 55% of STS participant sites did fewer than five esophagectomies per year. In 2016, the lung cancer resection risk model was also updated.[15] Again, three hierarchical logistic regression models were created to estimate the association of patient characteristics with the outcomes of mortality, major morbidity, and the composite of both. Between January 1, 2012, and December 31, 2014, there were 27,844 lung cancer resections in the database from 231 centers. Mortality was down to 1.4%, whereas major morbidity was 9.1% and the composite 9.5%. Variation in hospital performance in the composite measure was also examined by using a Bayesian approach to compute standardized incidence ratios with 95% credible intervals for each hospital. This approach, again, allowed for discrimination between those centers performing better or worse than expected.

OPPORTUNITIES

The STS has developed several composite performance measures for adult cardiac surgery, including coronary artery bypass surgery, aortic valve replacement, and coronary artery bypass surgery plus aortic valve replacement.[16–18] All of these measures are publically reported and endorsed by the NQF.[6,19] The STS has recently developed a composite score for rating program performance for lobectomy for lung cancer and after it becomes publically reported, may be an excellent measure for endorsement at the NQF.[20] Similar to the adult cardiac composite measures, composite quality was based on observed to expected mortality and major complications rates after lung cancer resection. Participant-specific risk-adjusted rates of 30-day mortality and major morbidity were estimated in a Bayesian hierarchical model where mortality was weighted four times greater than complications. Participant-specific composite scores were then ranked with 95% credible intervals. Programs whose 95% credible interval was entirely lower than the STS average were given one star (n = 8; 4.7%) and those that were entirely higher than the STS average were given three stars (n = 12; 7%). Two stars, the expected outcome for a database participant, were given to those programs whose credible interval overlapped the STS average.

Currently there are no measures addressing the appropriateness of surgery, the surgical approach, the oncologic efficacy of the surgery, or readmissions. These may represent further opportunities for measure development.

SUMMARY

The leadership of the STS has been at the forefront of development and maintenance of quality performance measures in thoracic surgery. The currently endorsed measures represent the only general thoracic surgery measures endorsed within the NQF. The measures include structure, process, and outcome measures and in time may include a publically reported composite measure. With the maturation of the general thoracic database, the addition of long-term follow-up, and the addition of readmission data, opportunities for further measure development abound.

REFERENCES

1. Hyder JA, Roy N, Wakeam E, et al. Performance measurement in surgery through the National Quality Forum. J Am Coll Surg 2014;219:1037–46.
2. The American Board of Surgery. Maintenance of Certification. Available at: http://www.absurgery.org/default.jsp?exam-mocreqs. Accessed October 30, 2016.
3. The American Board of Thoracic Surgery. Maintenance of Certification. Available at: https://www.abts.org/root/home/maintenance-of-certification-(moc).aspx. Accessed October 30, 2016.
4. CMS. Available at: https://www.cms.gov/Medicare/Quality-Initiatives-Patient-Assessment-Instruments/hospital-value-based-purchasing/index.html. Accessed October 30, 2016.
5. Jacobs JP, Shahian DM, Prager RL, et al. Introduction to the STS National Database Series: Outcomes Analysis, Quality Improvement, and Patient Safety. Ann Thorac Surg 2015;100:1992–2000.
6. National Quality Forum. Available at: https://www.qualityforum.org/. Accessed October 13, 2016.
7. Kizer KW. Patient safety: a call to action: a consensus statement from the National Quality Forum. MedGenMed 2001;3(2):10.
8. Bester H. Quality uncertainty mitigates product differentiation. Rand J Econ 1998;29(4):828–44.
9. Chassin MR, Galvin RW. The urgent need to improve health care quality: Institute of Medicine National Roundtable on Health Care Quality. JAMA 1998;280(11):1000–5.
10. Kizer KW. The National Quality Forum seeks to improve health care. Acad Med 2000;76(4):320–1.
11. Miller T, Leatherman S. The National Quality Forum: a 'Me-Too' or a breakthrough in quality measurement and reporting. Health Aff 1999;18(6):233–7.
12. Wright CD, Gaissert HA, Grab JD, et al. Predictors of prolonged length of stay after lobectomy for lung cancer: a Society of Thoracic Surgeons General Thoracic Surgery Database risk-adjusted model. Ann Thorac Surg 2008;85:1857–65.
13. Wright CD, Kucharczuk JC, O'Brien SM, et al. Predictors of major morbidity and mortality after esophagectomy for esophageal cancer: a Society of Thoracic Surgeons General Thoracic Surgery Database risk adjusted model. J Thorac Cardiovasc Surg 2009;137:587–96.
14. Kozower BD, Sheng S, O'Brien SM, et al. STS database risk models: predictors of mortality and major morbidity for lung cancer resection. Ann Thorac Surg 2010;90:875–83.
15. Fernandez FG, Kosinski AS, Burfeind WR, et al. The Society of Thoracic Surgeons lung cancer resection risk model: higher quality data and superior outcomes. Ann Thorac Surg 2016;102:370–7.
16. Shahian DM, O'Brien SM, Filardo G, et al. The Society of Thoracic Surgeons 2008 cardiac surgery risk models: part 1-coronary artery bypass grafting surgery. Ann Thorac Surg 2009;88(Suppl):2–22.
17. Shahian DM, He X, Jacobs JP, et al. The Society of Thoracic Surgeons isolated aortic valve replacement (AVR) composite score: a report of the STS Quality Measurement Task Force. Ann Thorac Surg 2012;94:2166–71.
18. Shahian DM, He X, Jacobs JP, et al. The STS AVR + CABG composite score: a report of the STS Quality Measurement Task Force. Ann Thorac Surg 2014;97:1604–9.
19. The Society of Thoracic Surgeons. Public Reporting. Available at: http://www.sts.org/quality-research-patient-safety/sts-public-reporting-online. Accessed October 30, 2016.
20. Kozower BD, O'Brien SM, Kosinski AS, et al. The Society of Thoracic Surgeons composite score for rating program performance for lobectomy for lung cancer. Ann Thorac Surg 2016;101:1379–87.

Volume-Outcome Relationships in Thoracic Surgery

Benjamin D. Kozower, MD, MPH[a],*,
George J. Stukenborg, PhD[b]

KEYWORDS

- Volume outcome • Thoracic surgery • Cancer resection • Lung cancer • Esophageal cancer

KEY POINTS

- Most thoracic surgery studies indicate that hospital and surgeon procedure volume are inversely associated with mortality.
- Controversy exists regarding the strength and validity of this volume-outcome association.
- Because thresholds of procedure volume are used to recommend the regionalization of care, investigation of the volume-outcome relationship is imperative.
- Careful examination of the literature demonstrates that lung and esophageal cancer resection volume is not strongly associated with mortality and should not be used as a proxy measure for quality.

INTRODUCTION

Surgeons and hospitals are under incredible pressure to improve the quality of care they deliver. However, debate exists regarding which outcomes measures should be used to reflect surgical quality.[1] Procedure volume has been studied as a predictor of surgical outcomes since Luft and colleagues[2] first promoted the volume-outcome relationship in 1979. Volume is an appealing predictor of surgical outcomes because it is easily measured, inexpensive, and because it makes intuitive sense. Higher-volume hospitals are more likely to have the structural and process measures in place to achieve better outcomes.[1] Most studies examining the volume-outcome relationship after lung cancer resection conclude that patients in hospitals with higher procedure volumes have significantly lower mortality risk.[3–6] These studies show a decrease of 1% to 4% in 30-day mortality rates between the highest- and lowest-volume centers.

Methodologic reviews of volume-outcome studies have noted serious concerns with the statistical methods used to identify this association.[7,8] Despite these concerns, procedure volume has been used to recommend the regionalization of surgical procedures using selected volume thresholds.[9] The volume-outcome association is complex, and debate continues as to how it should be used by public and private organizations caring for patients.[10,11] Furthermore, there are a range of unintended consequences that need to be considered if procedure volume is used to direct patient referrals and regionalize health care.[10]

EVIDENCE SUPPORTING THE VOLUME OUTCOME RELATIONSHIP IN LUNG CANCER RESECTION

The seminal article describing the relationship between increasing case volume and improved outcomes was published by Luft and colleagues[2] in 1979. They demonstrated that hospitals in which

[a] Washington University School of Medicine, 660 South Euclid Avenue, Campus Box 8234, St Louis, MO 63110, USA; [b] University of Virginia School of Medicine, PO Box 800717, Charlottesville, VA 22908, USA
* Corresponding author.
E-mail address: kozowerb@wudosis.wustl.edu

Thorac Surg Clin 27 (2017) 251–256
http://dx.doi.org/10.1016/j.thorsurg.2017.03.004

certain complicated operations were performed 200 or more times annually had case-adjusted death rates up to 41% lower than hospitals with lower volumes. Twenty years later, the interest in the volume-outcome association in lung cancer resection increased exponentially, led by publications from Birkmeyer and colleagues[3] and Bach and colleagues.[4] Bach and colleagues[4] investigated the volume-outcome relationship using patients from the linked Surveillance, Epidemiology, and End Results Program and Medicare Databases, and who underwent surgery in a hospital that participates in the Nationwide Inpatient Sample. This article was unique in that it looked at 5-year survival rather than in-hospital or 30-day survival. The authors divided volume into five groups (quintiles) and used traditional survival modeling techniques to examine the association between hospital procedure volume and survival. The article concluded that patients who undergo resection for lung cancer at the highest-volume hospitals had an 11% increase in 5-year survival and had lower complication rates. The following year (2002), Birkmeyer and colleagues[3] also published their findings on the volume-outcome relationship. Using data from Medicare claims and the Nationwide Inpatient Sample, they investigated the relationship between hospital procedure volume and 30-day mortality for 14 different procedures, including lung cancer resection. The authors also divided volume into arbitrarily defined categories and concluded that in the absence of other information about the quality of surgery at the hospitals near them, Medicare patients undergoing selected procedures can significantly reduce their risk of operative death by selecting a high-volume hospital.

Birkmeyer and colleagues[12] also demonstrated that surgeon volume is directly related to outcome. Using information from the national Medicare claims database, they examined mortality among 474,108 patients who underwent one of eight cardiovascular procedures or cancer resections. They demonstrated that surgeon volume was inversely related to operative mortality for all eight high-risk operative procedures, including lung cancer resection. The adjusted odds ratio for postoperative mortality for low-volume surgeons compared with high-volume surgeons was 1.24 for lung cancer resection. In addition, they demonstrated that much of the observed association between hospital volume and operative mortality was mediated by individual surgeon volume. The authors concluded that patients may be able to improve their chances of survival substantially, even at high-volume hospitals, by selecting surgeons who perform particular operations frequently.

METHODOLOGIC ISSUES WITH CURRENT EVIDENCE

There are serious methodologic concerns with the three landmark studies cited previously and most volume-outcome studies reported in the literature. First, most volume-outcome studies place procedure volumes into arbitrarily defined categories (tertiles, quartiles, quintiles), rather than treating volume as a continuous variable. This results in a loss of information and arbitrarily inflates the effect of volume on mortality risk when measured by odds ratios.[13] It also makes odds ratios difficult to compare from one study to the next because studies use different volume category partitioning. The preferred method for studying the relationship between procedure volume and mortality is to represent volume as a continuous variable and assess its linear and nonlinear relationships with mortality. This can best be accomplished using restricted cubic spline regression.[14,15] Spline regression creates a functional representation of the shape of the relationship between volume and the outcome of mortality using piecewise polynomial functions. Spline regression is the most accurate method to characterize nonlinearity present in the volume-outcome relationship, because it uses all the data points to estimate the shape of an association between an exposure (volume) and the outcome (mortality).[11,16–18] Unfortunately, most researchers are not familiar with this technique and have not used it to determine if a true threshold value exists for the volume-outcome relationship in lung cancer resection.

A second common problem is the use of traditional multivariable logistic regression models to test the significance of the relationship between procedure volume and inpatient mortality.[8,11] When the predictor variables include patient-level variables (age, sex, comorbidity) and hospital-level variables (procedure volume), it is essential to use multilevel modeling techniques, such as hierarchical generalized linear models. This modeling technique accounts for correlated outcomes within hospitals and adjusts for potentially overdispersed variance estimates. It is imperative that volume-outcome studies use hierarchical modeling, including hospitals as random effects in the models, to allow the relationship between volume and inpatient death to be different across hospitals.[19] Urbach and Austin[20] compared the use of conventional statistical models with multilevel regression models in volume-outcome analyses. They determined that the modeling techniques yield substantially different results, with conventional models overestimating the volume-outcome relationship. They concluded that conventional models should not be used for volume-outcome analyses of surgical procedures.

Another common problem is that most volume-outcome studies use administrative data sources containing an enormous number of surgical procedures. This increases the potential to observe a statistical significance in the relationship between volume and mortality without understanding the clinical significance.[8] Therefore, it is imperative to report the effect sizes and the relative importance of volume compared with other predictors of mortality.[21] In addition, the quality and performance of the statistical models used is frequently not reported. This is a crucial mistake because the point estimates and odds ratios need to be interpreted in the context of model performance. For example, the C statistic is equivalent to the area under the receiver operating characteristic curve for models with a dichotomous response variable, such as mortality (alive or dead). It provides an estimate of the model's ability to discriminate between observed instances of inpatient death and survival. A value of 0.5 indicates that the model provides no predictive discrimination, whereas a value of 1.0 indicates perfect separation. Importantly, if the C statistic for a model is 0.5, the point estimates and odds ratios for the different variables in the model are almost irrelevant, because the model performance is so poor.

The final methodologic issue discussed in this article is the importance of proper risk adjustment. In 1997, the Veterans Affairs (VA) administration considered closing low-volume centers to decrease cost and improve outcome.[22] To determine the feasibility of this plan, the National Surgical Quality Improvement Program (NSQIP) examined the relationship of surgical volume to outcome in eight common operations.[23] Four different types of statistical analyses showed no relationship between the 30-day mortality observed/expected ratio and procedure volume in any of the eight operations examined. In fact, in this study, the hospital with the highest volume of colectomies was one of the three outliers in the 22-hospital system and a hospital in the lower quartile for volume had the lowest mortality. In the face of these compelling data, managers in the VA system did not institute the volume-based system. Why did this VA study contradict the intuitive findings of other volume-outcome studies? The use of clinical rather than administrative data in previous studies supporting the volume-outcome relationship is crucial because administrative data have limited ability to differentiate comorbidity, severity of illness, and case mix.[24–26] This may contribute to selection bias in studies using administrative

data because patient risk factors were not accounted for in many earlier studies. Importantly, the risk adjustment of administrative data has significantly improved, but is not used in most volume-outcome studies.

The most effective system for risk-adjusting administrative data was developed by Elixhauser and colleagues.[27] It uses 30 categories of comorbidity measures and is used by the Agency for Healthcare Research and Quality. The comorbidities were associated with substantial increases in length of stay, hospital charges, and mortality for heterogeneous and homogeneous disease groups. Several comorbidities are described that are important predictors of outcomes, yet commonly are not measured. The Elixhauser method has been demonstrated to provide effective adjustments for mortality risk among surgical populations.[28,29]

THORACIC SURGERY VOLUME-OUTCOME STUDIES ADDRESSING METHODOLOGIC CONCERNS

Stukenborg and colleagues[16] evaluated temporal order and nonlinearity in the relationship between lung cancer resection volume and in-hospital mortality. They examined this relationship using 14,456 California hospital patients from 330 hospitals. Restricted cubic splines were used to model the nonlinearity of the volume-outcome relationship, and the authors found that large decreases in procedure volume were associated with very small absolute increases in mortality risk. They also found that the volume of lung cancer operations during the year before a patient's admission was not a statistically significant predictor of mortality after lung cancer resection. To improve the risk-adjustment of administrative data, Stukenborg and colleagues[30] used present-at-admission diagnoses in another study of the volume-outcome relationship in lung cancer. Importantly, this technique improved the performance characteristics of their model compared with other risk adjustment strategies using administrative data, which did not take the present-at-admission diagnoses into account.

The relationship between hospital lung cancer resection volume and in-hospital mortality was recently evaluated using three methods for measuring the effect of volume.[31] The study used the Nationwide Inpatient Sample database because it is the largest all-payer inpatient database available in the United States, representing a 20% sample of all hospital discharges from nonfederal facilities.[32] They evaluated 40,460 lung cancer resection patients, and volume was empirically assessed as a linear variable, as a nonlinear variable using arbitrarily selected quintile categories, and using restricted cubic spline regression. Importantly, hierarchical modeling was used to account for the multilevel data, and they reported model performance characteristics along with the relative importance of hospital procedure volume compared with other predictors of mortality. In addition, the Elixhauser method was used to risk-adjust these administrative data. Their results demonstrated that hospital lung cancer resection volume was a statistically significant predictor of mortality when measured using quintiles (odds ratio, 3.52) but not when represented as a linear variable or when using restricted cubic spline regression. These analyses demonstrated how categorization of the volume variable can artificially inflate the odds ratio and the apparent importance of volume as a predicator of mortality. However, when they assessed the importance of volume compared with other predictors of mortality, even in the model representing volume as quintiles, the relative contribution of volume for predicting mortality was small compared with patient age and comorbidities. Importantly, the authors reported excellent model performance with a C statistic of 0.92. This article concluded that the impact of procedure volume on mortality depends on how volume is represented and that the use of volume as a proxy measure for quality is problematic.

The Society of Thoracic Surgeons (STS) General Thoracic Surgery Database is a detailed specialty based database that captures 30-day outcomes after thoracic surgery. Wright and colleagues[33] used these data to evaluate the volume-outcome relationship in esophageal cancer resection. Despite this database consisting of primarily general thoracic surgeons, esophagectomy volume ranged from 1 to 83 with most hospitals performing fewer than 10 procedures per year. This STS national study using detailed clinical data found no association between esophagectomy volume and a composite outcome of morbidity and mortality. It concluded that volume is an inadequate proxy for quality assessment after esophagectomy.

Another recent volume-outcome analysis in thoracic surgery reported on survival differences after lung transplantation.[34] This study used data from the United Network for Organ Sharing registry for 15,642 adult lung transplantation patients from 61 centers in the United States. Their primary objective was to assess variability in long-term survival after lung transplantation among hospitals in the United States. They identified a weak volume-outcome relationship, but

significant variability in hospital performance remained, after controlling for procedure volume. The authors concluded that further exploration of the causes of hospital variation is warranted because presumed predictors of outcome do not explain large amounts of the variability between hospitals.

QUALITY MEASUREMENT

This article seems to contradict the adage that "practice makes perfect." Lung cancer resection is a fairly high-risk procedure with a current in-hospital mortality of between 2% and 3%.[31,35] Many surgeons, patients, and policy makers believe that the risk of mortality with complicated surgical procedures decreases with increased hospital and surgeon volume. However, most studies examining the volume-outcome relationship have measured the effects of volume using arbitrary categorization, inappropriate statistical modeling techniques, and inadequate risk adjustment, and typically fail to provide information about the relative contribution of volume compared with other predictors of mortality.[8] Hospital and surgeon volume are only a proxy for the multidimensional concept of institutional experience.[36] There are unmeasured, unknown factors at a hospital level that have a much greater influence on mortality than volume.[34]

Surgeons would like to believe that they, and not the government or insurance industry, should set the standards for surgical care. It is crucial that surgeons participate in the development of accurate clinical databases and risk-adjusted data. The NSQIP program was an excellent start, but a tremendous difference exists between the VA system and the rest of American surgery. The VA was able to insist on mandatory reporting and designed a risk-adjustment system. The government pays to train the data coordinators and for independent audits. They have a good electronic medical record that helps with data collection. The VA centers have protected communication between them, and the VA has created an environment where the data were used to improve quality rather than penalize poor performers. The NSQIP program is indeed an excellent example of surgeons directing the quality of surgical care.

In an effort for general thoracic surgeons to direct quality assessment, the STS General Thoracic Surgery Database was initiated in 2002. The STS Cardiac Surgery Database is the gold standard for clinical data analysis registries. It has been instrumental in determining risk-adjusted outcome measures and influencing public policy.[37] The General Thoracic Surgery Database is only in its infancy, but it continues to grow and to illustrate the understanding that surgeons have for setting their own benchmarks based on accurate detailed clinical data. The database was recently used to study hospital performance variation in lung cancer resection using a composite measure of mortality and major morbidity.[35] They reported on more than 27,000 lung cancer resections performed at 231 hospitals and found that there were statistically significant differences between the best and worst performing hospitals. However, the predictors of improved hospital performance are poorly understood and have not been further investigated. The use of clinical outcomes data to document quality is expensive and time consuming, but surgeons and hospitals deserve to be judged by their outcomes, not an arbitrary proxy for quality, such as a volume threshold.

A major issue with the use of volume as an indicator of quality is the problem of sample size. The Agency for Healthcare Research and Quality advocated that mortality should be an indicator of quality for seven major operations.[38] However, many of these procedures are performed infrequently at individual hospitals and mortality rates for a given procedure can have large variations. Therefore, it may be difficult to identify a difference in mortality rates based on volume. Dimick and colleagues[38] evaluated this issue by looking at the proportion of hospitals in the United States that perform enough of these seven high-risk procedures to accurately detect a doubling in the mortality rate. They concluded that, with the exception of coronary artery bypass grafting, the procedures for which surgical mortality has been advocated as a quality indicator are not performed frequently enough to detect a doubling in the mortality rate.

It needs to be asked if thoracic surgeons and the STS National Database are adequately measuring quality.[10] Surgeons have done a remarkable job recording and improving on their 30-day outcomes. However, documenting long-term follow-up and incorporating meaningful measures of functional outcomes and quality of life have been more difficult. The current data points in surgical registries do not reflect patient and family satisfaction or the quality of life after procedures. This enormously important information continues to lag behind other quality improvement initiatives. It is imperative that the thoracic surgery community incorporates these outcomes measures into an accurate clinical database that enables physicians and patients to make informed decisions and accurately assess quality.

SUMMARY

Further research is required to determine whether volume-based regionalization of thoracic surgery improves the quality of surgical care in the United States. The volume-outcome relationship is extremely complicated, and the financial and ethical implications of a volume-based referral strategy are equally complex.[10,11] The large volume-outcome relationship that was initially demonstrated using administrative data with serious methodologic concerns has disappeared with the use of accurate clinical data, better risk-adjustment of administrative data, and more accurate statistical methods for evaluating the volume-outcome relationship. It is imperative that health care providers be measured on their outcomes and that the large group of stakeholders examining the volume-outcome relationship understand that it is a poor proxy measure for quality.

REFERENCES

1. Birkmeyer JD, Dimick JB, Birkmeyer NJ. Measuring the quality of surgical care: structure, process, or outcomes? J Am Coll Surg 2004;198:626–32.
2. Luft HS, Bunker JP, Enthoven AC. Should operations be regionalized? The empirical relation between surgical volume and mortality. N Engl J Med 1979;301: 1364–9.
3. Birkmeyer JD, Siewers AE, Finlayson EV, et al. Hospital volume and surgical mortality in the United States. N Engl J Med 2002;346:1128–37.
4. Bach PB, Cramer LD, Schrag D, et al. The influence of hospital volume on survival after resection for lung cancer. N Engl J Med 2001;345:181–8.
5. Romano PS, Mark DH. Patient and hospital characteristics related to in-hospital mortality after lung cancer resection. Chest 1992;101:1332–7.
6. Finlayson EV, Goodney PP, Birkmeyer JD. Hospital volume and operative mortality in cancer surgery: a national study. Arch Surg 2003;138:721–5.
7. Halm EA, Lee C, Chassin MR. Is volume related to outcome in health care? A systematic review and methodologic critique of the literature. Ann Intern Med 2002;137:511–20.
8. Livingston EH, Cao J. Procedure volume as a predictor of surgical outcomes. JAMA 2010;304:95–7.
9. Leapfrog G. Evidence-based hospital referral. Available at: http://www.leapfroggroup.org/media/file/ Leapfrog-Evidence-Based_Hospital_ Referral_Fact_ Sheet.pdf. Accessed October 12, 2016.
10. Kozower BD, Stukenborg GJ, Lau CL, et al. Measuring the quality of surgical outcomes in general thoracic surgery: should surgical volume be used to direct patient referrals? Ann Thorac Surg 2008;86:1405–8.

11. Shahian DM, Normand SL. The volume-outcome relationship: from Luft to leapfrog. Ann Thorac Surg 2003;75:1048–58.

12. Birkmeyer JD, Stukel TA, Siewers AE, et al. Surgeon volume and operative mortality in the United States. N Engl J Med 2003;349:2117–27.

13. Royston P, Altman DG, Sauerbrei W. Dichotomizing continuous predictors in multiple regression: a bad idea. Stat Med 2006;25:127–41.

14. Rosenberg PS, Katki H, Swanson CA, et al. Quantifying epidemiologic risk factors using nonparametric regression: model selection remains the greatest challenge. Stat Med 2003;22:3369–81.

15. Harrell FE Jr, Lee KL, Pollock BG. Regression models in clinical studies: determining relationships between predictors and response. J Natl Cancer Inst 1988;80:1198–202.

16. Stukenborg GJ, Wagner DP, Harrell FE. Temporal order and nonlinearity in the relationship between lung cancer resection volume and in-hospital mortality. Health Serv Outcomes Res Methodol 2004;5:59–73.

17. Greenland S. Avoiding power loss associated with categorization and ordinal scores in dose response and trend analysis. Epidemiology 1995;6:450–4.

18. Greenland S. Dose-response and trend analysis in epidemiology: alternatives to categorical analysis. Epidemiology 1995;6:356–65.

19. Panageas KS, Schrag D, Riedel E, et al. The effect of clustering of outcomes on the association of procedure volume and surgical outcomes. Ann Intern Med 2003;139:658–65.

20. Urbach DR, Austin PC. Conventional models overestimate the statistical significance of volume-outcome associations, compared with multilevel models. J Clin Epidemiol 2005;58:391–400.

21. Livingston EH, Elliot A, Hynan L, et al. Effect size estimation: a necessary component of statistical analysis. Arch Surg 2009;144:706–12.

22. Khuri SF. Quality, advocacy, healthcare policy, and the surgeon. Ann Thorac Surg 2002;74:641–9.

23. Khuri SF, Daley J, Henderson W, et al. Relation of surgical volume to outcome in eight common operations: results from the VA National Surgical Quality Improvement Program. Ann Surg 1999;230:414–29.

24. Hsia DC. Accuracy of Medicare reimbursement for cardiac arrest. JAMA 1990;264:59–62.

25. Fisher ES, Whaley FS, Krushat WM, et al. The accuracy of Medicare's hospital claims data: progress has been made, but problems remain. Am J Public Health 1992;82:243–8.

26. Iezzoni LI, Foley SM, Daley J, et al. Comorbidities, complications, and coding bias. Does the number of diagnosis codes matter in predicting in-hospital mortality? JAMA 1992;267:2197–203.

27. Elixhauser A, Steiner C, Harris DR, et al. Comorbidity measures for use with administrative data. Med Care 1990;36:8–27.

28. Southern DA, Quan H, Ghali WA. Comparison of the Elixhauser and Charlson/Deyo methods of comorbidity measurement in administrative data. Med Care 2004;42:355–60.

29. Stukenborg GJ, Wagner DP, Connors AF Jr. Comparison of the performance of two comorbidity measures, with and without information from prior hospitalizations. Med Care 2001;39:727–39.

30. Stukenborg GJ, Kilbridge KL, Wagner DP, et al. Present-at-admission diagnoses improve mortality risk adjustment and allow more accurate assessment of the relationship between volume of lung cancer operations and mortality risk. Surgery 2005;138:498–507.

31. Kozower BD, Stukenborg GJ. The relationship between hospital lung cancer resection volume and patient mortality risk. Ann Surg 2011;254:1032–7.

32. Nationwide inpatient sample. Available at: http://www.hcup-us.ahrq.gov/nisoverview.jsp. Accessed September 30, 2016.

33. Wright CD, Kucharczuk JC, O'Brien SM, et al. Predictors of major morbidity and mortality after esophagectomy for esophageal cancer: a Society of Thoracic Surgeons General Thoracic Surgery Database risk adjustment model. J Thorac Cardiovasc Surg 2009;137:587–95.

34. Thabut G, Christie JD, Kremers WK, et al. Survival differences following lung transplantation among US transplant centers. JAMA 2010;304:53–60.

35. Fernandez FG, Kosinski AS, Burfeind W, et al. The Society of Thoracic Surgeons Lung Cancer Resection Risk Model: Higher Quality Data and Superior Outcomes. Ann Thorac Surg 2016;102:370–7.

36. Hannan EL. The relation between volume and outcome in health care. N Engl J Med 1999;340:1677–9.

37. Shahian DM, Edwards FH, Ferraris VA, et al. Quality measurement in adult cardiac surgery: part 1—Conceptual framework and measure selection. Ann Thorac Surg 2007;83(4 suppl):S3–12.

38. Dimick JB, Welch HG, Birkmeyer JD. Surgical mortality as an indicator of hospital quality: the problem with small sample size. JAMA 2004;292:847–51.

Failure-to-Rescue in Thoracic Surgery

Farhood Farjah, MD, MPH

KEYWORDS

- Failure-to-rescue • Quality improvement • Thoracic surgery

KEY POINTS

- Failure-to-rescue is defined as death during hospitalization among patients who experience a complication.
- Failure-to-rescue is best measured using a clinical registry that allows for robust risk adjustment and accurate ascertainment of postoperative complications.
- Failure-to-rescue explains a greater degree of variability in hospital-level mortality compared with complications.
- Preventing complications and rescue will likely reduce the number of untimely deaths after thoracic surgery.

INTRODUCTION

Variation in the safety and effectiveness of care has led to a sustained interest in improving the quality of thoracic surgical care.[1–7] Using Avedis Donabedian's framework of outcome, process, and structure,[8] leaders within this field have proposed improving quality through a variety of interventions, including performance feedback measured in terms of risk-adjusted short-term outcomes,[9] process compliance,[10] and regionalization of care based on surgeon specialty or volume.[1–3,5,6] Despite these well-intended efforts, our knowledge of drivers of quality remains limited. Therefore, our ability to improve quality is also limited.

In the early 1990s, Silber and colleagues[11] set out to better understand the mechanisms underlying early death after surgery. They found that rescuing patients from complications explained more of the variability in early death rates than did preventing complications. This work is significant because it challenged conventional wisdom focusing predominantly on preventing complications. This article highlights key concepts

surrounding failure-to-rescue and reviews the literature on failure-to-rescue in noncardiac thoracic surgery.

BRIEF HISTORY

Dr Silber hypothesized that factors associated with complications are different from factors associated with rescuing patients with complications. Specifically, he believed that patient characteristics drive complication rates, whereas hospital characteristics drive rescue. Using administrative data provided by the Health Care Financing Administration, Silber and colleagues[11] studied patients who underwent cholecystectomy or transurethral prostatectomy across 7 states in the 1980s. They evaluated whether a relationship existed between patient-specific (eg, age, severity of illness) and hospital-specific characteristics (eg, board-certified surgeons, trainees) and 3 different outcomes—death, complications, and failure-to-rescue (defined as death among patients with a complication). In general, patient characteristics were associated with complications, whereas

The author has nothing to disclose.
Megan Zadworny, MHA assisted greatly in the preparation of this article.
Division of Cardiothoracic Surgery, University of Washington, 1959 Northeast Pacific Street, Box 356310, Seattle, WA 98195, USA
E-mail address: ffarjah@uw.edu

Thorac Surg Clin 27 (2017) 257–266
http://dx.doi.org/10.1016/j.thorsurg.2017.03.005
1547-4127/17/© 2017 Elsevier Inc. All rights reserved.

hospital characteristics were associated with failure-to-rescue. Having found evidence to support their theory, the authors proposed measuring death, complication, and failure-to-rescue rates with an eye toward allowing hospital managers to direct resources as needed to the areas of greatest concern (eg, prevention, rescue, or both).

Critics of Dr Silber's suggested that administrative data are inaccurate for measuring complications and have insufficient granularity to allow for robust risk adjustment.[12,13] To address this concern, a group of researchers from the University of Michigan used a clinical registry maintained by the American College of Surgeons National Surgical Quality Improvement Program (ACS-NSQIP) to study failure-to-rescue after general and vascular surgical procedures.[14] Their analysis was slightly different than that of that of Dr Silber's group. Ghaferi and associates[14] ranked hospitals according to their risk-adjusted mortality rates and then compared rates of complications and failure-to-rescue across these rankings. Complication rates did not vary significantly across hospitals, but failure-to-rescue rates did. Similar to Dr Silber's work, these findings suggest that failure-to-rescue was a greater driver of surgical mortality than prevention of complications.

A result of this early work is that both the Agency for Healthcare Research and Quality and the National Quality Forum now endorse failure-to-rescue as a hospital-level quality metric.[15,16]

CONCEPTUAL FRAMEWORK

Failure-to-rescue is an outcome that measures safety. It is not an intuitive metric, perhaps because the numerator for both failure-to-rescue and operative mortality are both death. For this reason, it is not possible to analyze the relationship between failure-to-rescue and death in the same way one would study the relationship between

volume and outcome using regression or thoracoscopy and outcomes using propensity scores. One way to conceptualize failure-to-rescue is to consider it a mechanism by which patients die in the early postoperative period. It is an intermediate outcome in the causal pathway linking an operation to inpatient survival or death (Fig. 1).

Causes of Early Death After Thoracic Surgery

Almost all patients who die in the early postoperative period do so because of a complication. Other causes of inpatient death are suicide or homicide. A recent literature review spanning 26 years reported 335 reported cases of inpatient suicide in the nonpsychiatric hospitalized setting.[17] The Bureau for Labor Statistics reported 17 homicides in the health care setting between 1997 and 2010[18] and the Joint Commissions Sentinel Event Database reported 22 patient homicides between 2010 and 2014.[19] Although inpatient suicide and homicide are important safety concerns, the rarity of these events and impracticality of measuring them leads us to reasonably assume—for the purposes of measuring failure-to-rescue—that all inpatient deaths after surgery are caused by complications.

Ways to Avoid Early Death After Thoracic Surgery

If all early deaths after thoracic surgery are caused by complications, then there are 2 distinct ways to avoid death: (1) prevent complications from occurring or (2) rescue patients who have a complication (see Fig. 1). Most interventions designed by thoracic surgeons aim to prevent postoperative complications. For instance, minimally invasive approaches to pulmonary resection and esophagectomy are intended to reduce the incidence of complications.[20,21] Likewise, chemoprophylaxis reduces the incidence of postoperative atrial

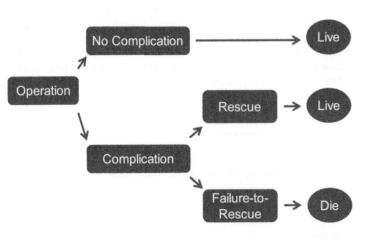

Fig. 1. Conceptual framework for death after an operation.

fibrillation after major noncardiac thoracic surgery.[22–25] There are no published examples of interventions designed by thoracic surgeons that explicitly aim to rescue patients form early death.

Ways to Rescue Patients from Early Death After Thoracic Surgery

There are 3 potential ways to rescue patients from an early death after thoracic surgery: (1) detect complications early, (2) treat complications early, or (3) detect and treat complications early. Early detection may allow one to treat a complication when it is in a more treatable (ie, less severe) form. There are 2 ways in which early treatment may be beneficial. Early treatment can mitigate the severity of a complication. For instance, early and aggressive treatment of postoperative pneumonitis in a hypoxic patient supported with supplemental oxygen may help avoid progression toward a more severe manifestation requiring intubation and ventilator dependence. Early treatment of complications can prevent other associated complications that could cause a cascade toward death. For example, early treatment of postoperative pneumonitis and associated mild hypoxia may help avoid the development of atrial arrhythmias. Researchers using the Veteran's Affairs Surgical Quality Improvement Program database studied failure-to-rescue using the number of complications to investigate a potential dose-response relationship.[26] These investigators found that failure-to-rescue rates were higher among patients with an increasing number of complications. This finding is consistent with the idea that failure-to-rescue leads to cascading events. More likely than not, rescue depends on both early detection and treatment of postoperative complications.

Finding Empirical Evidence to Support Prevention or Rescue

To develop interventions that decrease mortality, we must understand the relative contributions of prevention and rescue to untimely deaths. **Fig. 2** shows hypothetical results for 3 different scenarios that explain early death after thoracic surgery. This hypothetical analysis is based on a contemporary approach to understanding the cause of death after surgery.[14,27] The first step is to rank order hospitals on the x-axis based on their risk-adjusted mortality rates (best to worst going left to right). Doing so allows us to compare hospital performance after accounting for potential differences in case mix. The second step is to compare complication rates across hospitals ranked by their risk-adjusted mortality rates. The third step is to compare failure-to-rescue rates across hospitals ranked by their risk-adjusted mortality rates.

Scenario A shows that complication rates are higher at higher-mortality hospitals, whereas failure-to-rescue rates do not vary across hospitals. These findings would support the hypothesis that prevention rather than rescue explains hospital-level variability in operative mortality rates. Scenario B shows that complication rates are invariant across hospitals ranked by risk-adjust mortality but that failure-to-rescue rates are higher at higher-mortality hospitals. These findings would support the hypothesis that rescue rather than prevention explains hospital-level variability in operative mortality rates. Scenario C shows that complication and failure-to-rescue rates are both higher among higher-mortality hospitals. These findings would support the hypothesis that both prevention and rescue are important. For some, these hypothetical results may not be intuitive when viewed graphically. **Table 1** shows the hypothetical results for 3 different hospitals in tabular form.

Potential Implications of Failure-to-Rescue Research

Failure-to-rescue research could redirect quality improvement interventions or serve as a metric for comparing hospital performance. As stated earlier, most existing interventions are directed toward preventing complications rather than rescuing patients from them. If research supports a more dominant influence of rescue on operative mortality, then that finding should lead us to design novel, system-level interventions directed toward the early detection and treatment of postoperative complications. Such findings would not preclude efforts to prevent complication but would direct more resources toward rescue. Because failure-to-rescue is an outcome measure, it could also be used to provide centers feedback about their performance. This information would not replace feedback on complication rates or risk-adjusted mortality rates. Instead, centers would have the opportunity to view their performance with regard to overall mortality, prevention, and rescue relative to their peers or a population benchmark. This information could allow centers to preferentially direct resources toward prevention or rescue tailored to specific performance gaps.

MEASUREMENT

Failure-to-rescue was originally defined as the probability of death after surgery given a complication.[11] Stated differently, failure-to-rescue is a proportion in which the numerator equals the number of deaths during the index hospitalization for

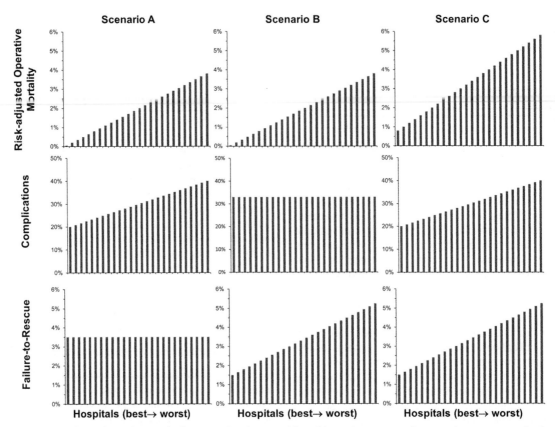

Fig. 2. Hypothetical graphic results for scenarios that provide evidence in support of prevention, rescue, or both. In these 3 hypothetical scenarios, hospitals are ranked according to their risk-adjusted operative mortality rates and ordered left to right from best to worst performance. Scenario A is one in which prevention is the only pathway by which one can mitigate the number of early deaths after thoracic surgery. In this scenario, one would observe significant variation in risk-adjusted operative mortality and complication rates. Failure-to-rescue rates would not vary across hospitals. Scenario B is one in which rescue is the only pathway by which one can mitigate the number of early deaths after thoracic surgery. In this scenario, one would observe significant variation in risk-adjusted operative mortality and failure-to-rescue rates. Complication rates would not vary across hospitals. Scenario C is one in which prevention and rescue are pathways by which one can mitigate the number of early deaths after thoracic surgery. In this scenario, one would observe significant variation in risk-adjusted operative mortality, complication, and failure-to-rescue rates.

Table 1
Hypothetical tabular results for scenarios that provide evidence in support of prevention, rescue, or both

	Scenario A			Scenario B			Scenario C		
	Hospital			Hospital			Hospital		
Raw Numbers	A	B	C	A	B	C	A	B	C
Patients	200	200	200	200	200	200	200	200	200
Complications	40	60	80	60	60	60	40	60	80
Deaths	2	3	4	2	3	4	1	3	5
Rates (%)									
Mortality	1.0	1.5	2.0	1.0	1.5	2.0	0.6	1.5	2.4
Complication	20	30	40	30	30	30	20	30	40
Failure-to-Rescue	5.0	5.0	5.0	3.3	5.0	6.7	3.0	5.0	6.3

surgery and the denominator equals the number patients with at least 1 complication. Subsequent to the first definition of failure-to-rescue emerged at least 2 others. One modification aimed to study deaths among patients with complications that could be detected early by nursing staff.[28] This definition included only 1 of at least 5 life-threatening complications: pneumonia, shock or cardiac arrest, upper gastrointestinal bleeding, sepsis, or deep venous thrombosis. Another modification, adopted by Agency for Healthcare Research and Quality, added renal failure to the list of nursing sensitive complications along with some other minor modifications.[29] These 2 alternative definitions were criticized for omitting 49% and 42% of all deaths that occur after general surgery and for having less reliability and validity compared with the original definition.[30]

With the emergence of clinical registries came slight modifications to the definition of failure-to-rescue. Clinical registries allow for more reliable and accurate assessment of postoperative complications. Audits of the ACS-NSQIP database and the Society of Thoracic Surgeons General Thoracic Surgery Database (STS-GTSD) found high reliability, accuracy, and completeness for both datasets.[31,32] In their study of general and vascular surgery, Ghaferi and colleagues[14] used the following events to define complications: superficial, deep, and organ-space infections; acute renal failure; postoperative bleeding requiring transfusion; myocardial infarction; pneumonia; pulmonary embolism; stroke; unplanned intubation; fascial dehiscence; prolonged mechanical ventilation (>48 h); deep venous thrombosis; urinary tract infection; septic shock; vascular graft loss; and renal insufficiency. Our research team used the STS-GTSD to study pulmonary resection and included any complication recorded by the registry to define failure-to-rescue.[27]

Failure-to-rescue has been repeatedly observed across operations regardless of the definitions or datasets used by investigators.[11,14,27,33–52] Based on the work by Silber and associates,[30] failure-to-rescue is best defined by the probability of death among patients who experience any postoperative complication. Ideally, failure-to-rescue studies should use clinical registry data that allows for robust risk-adjustment and accurate ascertainment of postoperative complications. However, one reason to use administrative datasets is to increase the generalizability of the findings to populations of patients and providers beyond those included in clinical registries. Another reason to use administrative data is to study the relationship between provider and hospital characteristics and failure-to-rescue. Most clinical registries collect

limited, if any, data on provider and hospital characteristics; if they do collect the data, they seldom release this information to researchers.

FAILURE-TO-RESCUE AND PULMONARY RESECTION

A PubMed search was performed on October 30, 2016 using the search term "failure-to-rescue AND (lung resection OR pulmonary resection OR lobectomy OR pneumonectomy OR lung cancer OR thoracic)." Twenty-seven articles were found. Thirteen studies included patients undergoing lung resection, albeit mixed with other patient populations.[26,27,33–43] Two studies examined failure-to-rescue among resected lung cancer patients,[27,33] whereas 1 investigation used failure-to-rescue to study the relationship between teaching hospitals and short-term outcomes.[41]

Our research team examined failure-to-rescue among resected lung cancer patients using the STS-GTSD clinical registry.[27] This study evaluated 30,000 patients across 208 institutions between 2009 and 2012. Hospitals were ranked by risk-adjusted mortality rates revealing 4-fold variation in the rates of early death among Society of Thoracic Surgeons participants. Complication rates varied across hospitals by approximately 20%, whereas failure-to-rescue rates varied by greater than 400%. These findings support the idea that rescue is the dominant factor leading to early death after lung resection.

A subsequent study using the National Cancer Database examined 645 lung resections performed at 43 hospitals among 645 patients between 2005 and 2006.[33] This study was unique in that it restricted the analysis to patients cared for at the highest and lowest risk–adjusted mortality hospitals (omitting intermediate-risk patients) and hospitals willing to participate in the study. The authors found no evidence of significant variation in complication rates across high and low risk–adjusted mortality hospitals, but they found evidence of considerable variation in failure-to-rescue rates.

Finally, a study evaluated the relationship between hospitals with thoracic surgery residency programs and short-term outcomes, one of which was failure-to-rescue.[41] This group linked the National Inpatient Sample to the American Hospital Association databases to determine which hospitals had thoracic surgery residency programs (vs general surgery or no training programs). Between 2003 and 2009, 498,099 patients were studied across 5585 hospitals. Compared with all other types of hospitals, those with thoracic surgery residency training programs were associated with lower complication, failure-to-rescue, and operative mortality rates.

FAILURE-TO-RESCUE AND ESOPHAGECTOMY

A PubMed search was performed on October 30, 2016 using the search term "failure-to-rescue AND (esophagectomy OR esophageal cancer OR thoracic)." Twenty-seven articles were found. Fourteen studies included patients undergoing esophagectomy, again mixed with other patient populations.[26,34,38–40,42–50] One study speculated on rescue as an explanation for the low mortality rate (0.5%) at a single center performing 200 transhiatal esophagectomies over 14 years.[45] The other investigation focused solely on esophagectomy and used failure-to-rescue to compare short-term outcomes across surgeon specialty.[47] The researchers used the National Inpatient Sample to study 23,529 esophagectomies performed between 1998 and 2008. They used surgeon case mix—defined as ≥65% of the operative case load consisting of cardiac, thoracic, or general surgical procedures—as a surrogate for surgeon subspecialty. Surgeons whose case load did not consist of ≥65% of one set of procedures were all grouped together as controls. The researchers reported that adjusted complication rates did not vary by surgeon subspecialty, but general surgeons were associated with higher mortality and failure-to-rescue rates compared with controls.

SIGNIFICANCE OF THE RESEARCH FINDINGS

The few available studies in noncardiac thoracic surgery show that variability in risk-adjusted mortality across hospitals is explained predominantly by a hospital's ability to rescue patients who experience a complication. This finding mirrors the literature examining general, vascular, adult cardiac, and congenital heart surgery.[14,51,52] However, unlike prior studies, which almost uniformly show that hospitals are equally good at preventing complications, our STS-GTSD analysis of pulmonary resection provided evidence to the contrary.[27] Some of the variation in hospital-level mortality rates is explained by the fact that some hospitals are better (or worse) at preventing complications. To the best of our knowledge, there is only one other study—of adult cardiac surgical patients—that reported a similar finding.[52] These findings are significant because they compel us to consider rescue strategies at least as often as—if not more often than—prevention strategies in our efforts to curb early death after thoracic surgery.

LIMITATIONS

One challenge with failure-to-rescue is distinguishing signal from noise in the context of performance measurement. Outcome measures can signal an opportunity to improve care if analysts can exclude the influence of case-mix and chance (ie, noise).[53] Clinical registries such as the STS-GTSD are well suited to collect information that allows for robust risk-adjustment. However, clinical registries cannot overcome the low volume of lung resections and esophagectomies (relative to other more frequently performed procedures such as coronary artery bypass grafting or colectomy).[54] Distinguishing signal from noise remains challenging, despite the availability of analytical techniques designed to mitigate the influence of chance.[55] The Society of Thoracic Surgeons has moved toward measuring surrogates for morbidity and mortality[56] or composite measures consisting of morbidity and mortality.[9] Indeed, when reviewers asked our research team to show evidence of outlier performance with regard to failure-to-rescue rate after pulmonary resection at a given hospital using the STS-GTSD, we were unable to do so with a reasonable level of statistical confidence.

Another limitation of failure-to-rescue is that system-level factors associated with it may not be modifiable. Factors such as nursing education and staffing,[57–59] hospital teaching and accreditation status,[30,41,43,60] payer mix,[61] bed size and daily census,[14] and the intensity of critical care services are associated with failure-to-rescue rates.[62] None of these factors are readily actionable. For instance, a nationwide shortage of nurses makes it challenging to increase staffing levels,[63] not to mention the increased associated costs of doing so. Debatably, the closest thing to a system-level intervention recently popularized by many hospitals and health systems is rapid response teams. Randomized trials failed to show reductions in early deaths attributable to either rapid response teams or validated, real-time automated systems that alert these teams.[64,65] Importantly, system-level interventions that work in the general inpatient setting may have no relevance to thoracic surgical patients.

POTENTIAL APPLICATIONS OF FAILURE-TO-RESCUE

One potential application of failure-to-rescue is to include complication and failure-to-rescue rates in performance reports as means of providing surgeons direction in improving early mortality.[11] Although not used to discern performance for the reasons provided earlier, information about complication and failure-to-rescue rates could help a surgeon leader to focus on prevention, rescue, or both as needed. A legitimate criticism of performance feedback measured in terms of risk-adjusted outcomes is that it does not provide direction on how to pursue quality improvement. Notably, 2 studies found that hospital participation in ACS-NSQIP had no association with outcomes, health care utilization, or costs.[66,67] Providing participants more granular information about the potential drivers of early mortality will help focus time, energy, and resources. Clinical registries that can provide participants all 3 outcome metrics—complication, failure-to-rescue, and early death rats—have an opportunity to lead performance measurement in a new direction.

Another application of measuring failure-to-rescue rates is to stimulate regional quality improvement collaboratives and other projects aimed at improving outcomes. Recent evidence of variability in outcomes, costs, and value across hospitals within a region further motivates such efforts.[7] Regional collaboratives have an opportunity to exchange information not readily measured by databases. For instance, the Michigan Society of Thoracic and Cardiovascular Surgery uses a phase of care mortality analysis as an opportunity to discover avoidable mortality triggers.[68] Their analysis of more than 1700 deaths found that 41% of deaths were avoidable and that just greater than 60% of avoidable deaths occurred because of triggers or seminal events in the hospital phase of care. Similar efforts decades earlier by the Northern New England Cardiovascular Disease Study Group learned that more than 70% of deaths were attributable to heart failure. Through this collaborative, system-level interventions designed to prevent and rescue patients from heart failure led to a 24% reduction in mortality rates across 8 hospitals in 2 years.[69,70]

Finally, the notion of failure-to-rescue could inspire young thoracic surgeons and investigators to develop system-level interventions aimed at rescuing patients. Historically, the focus of thoracic surgeons has been to prevent complications from occurring, for instance, through less-invasive surgery[20,21] or chemoprophylaxis for atrial arrhythmias.[22–24] System-level interventions might include protocols for early bronchoscopy to treat atelectasis, higher frequency surgeon rounding (including evenings), and continuous pulse oximetry and telemetry. An example of a policy-level intervention may include centralization of care to facilities staffed by board-certified thoracic surgeons. Prior findings show that lung cancer patients cared for by board-certified thoracic surgeons tend to have better short- and long-term outcomes and tend to receive recommended care more often.[5,6] Further evidence of a link between surgeon specialty and failure-to-rescue may strengthen the case to regionalize care based on surgeon characteristics.

SUMMARY

Failure-to-rescue is a quarter-century-old idea that invites us to think about early postoperative deaths differently. Prevention of complications will always remain our goal because (1) avoiding complications safeguards our patients from an untimely death and (2) complications cause suffering even if they do not lead to death. However, until we figure out how to reliably avoid complications associated with our high-risk operations, patients will continue to die. Although most thoracic surgeons likely believe in rescue, our history suggests that we have preferentially invested our resources in prevention. Perhaps that is why contemporary data show that our greatest opportunity for reducing untimely deaths is through system-level interventions that allow for early detection and treatment of postoperative complications.

REFERENCES

1. Birkmeyer JD, Siewers AE, Finlayson EV, et al. Hospital volume and surgical mortality in the United States. N Engl J Med 2002;346(15):1128–37.
2. Bach PB, Cramer LD, Schrag D, et al. The influence of hospital volume on survival after resection for lung cancer. N Engl J Med 2001;345(3):181–8.
3. Birkmeyer JD, Stukel TA, Siewers AE, et al. Surgeon volume and operative mortality in the United States. N Engl J Med 2003;349(22):2117–27.
4. Little AG, Rusch VW, Bonner JA, et al. Patterns of surgical care of lung cancer patients. Ann Thorac Surg 2005;80(6):2051–6 [discussion: 2056].
5. Goodney PP, Lucas FL, Stukel TA, et al. Surgeon specialty and operative mortality with lung resection. Ann Surg 2005;241(1):179–84.
6. Farjah F, Flum DR, Varghese TK Jr, et al. Surgeon specialty and long-term survival after pulmonary resection for lung cancer. Ann Thorac Surg 2009; 87(4):995–1004 [discussion: 1005–6].
7. Farjah F, Varghese TK, Costas K, et al. Lung resection outcomes and costs in Washington State: a case for regional quality improvement. Ann Thorac Surg 2014;98(1):175–81 [discussion: 182].
8. Donabedian A. Evaluating the quality of medical care. Milbank Mem Fund Q 1966;44(Suppl):166–206.
9. Fernandez FG, Kosinski AS, Burfeind W, et al. The Society of Thoracic Surgeons lung cancer resection

risk model: higher quality data and superior outcomes. Ann Thorac Surg 2016;102(2):370–7.

10. Katlic MR, Facktor MA, Berry SA, et al. ProvenCare lung cancer: a multi-institutional improvement collaborative. CA Cancer J Clin 2011;61(6):382–96.

11. Silber JH, Williams SV, Krakauer H, et al. Hospital and patient characteristics associated with death after surgery. A study of adverse occurrence and failure to rescue. Med Care 1992;30(7):615–29.

12. Romano PS, Chan BK, Schembri ME, et al. Can administrative data be used to compare postoperative complication rates across hospitals? Med Care 2002;40(10):856–67.

13. Lawson EH, Louie R, Zingmond DS, et al. A comparison of clinical registry versus administrative claims data for reporting of 30-day surgical complications. Ann Surg 2012;256(6):973–81.

14. Ghaferi AA, Birkmeyer JD, Dimick JB. Variation in hospital mortality associated with inpatient surgery. N Engl J Med 2009;361(14):1368–75.

15. Agency for Healthcare Research and Quality. Failure to rescue: percentage of patients who died with a complication in the hospital. 2015. Available at: https://www.qualitymeasures.ahrq.gov/summaries/summary/50111. Accessed October 29, 2016.

16. National Quality Forum. 2013. Available at: http://www.qualityforum.org/QPS. Accessed October 29, 2016.

17. Ballard ED, Pao M, Henderson D, et al. Suicide in the medical setting. Jt Comm J Qual Patient Saf 2008;34(8):474–81.

18. Bureau of Labor Statistics. Occupational homicides by selected characteristics: 1997-2010. Available at: http://www.bls.gov/iif/oshwc/cfoi/work_hom.pdf. Accessed October 29, 2016.

19. The Joint Commission. Preventing violent and criminal events. 2014. Available at: https://www.jointcommission.org/assets/1/23/Quick_Safety_Issue_Five_Aug_2014_FINAL.pdf. Accessed October 26, 2016.

20. Kirby TJ, Mack MJ, Landreneau RJ, et al. Lobectomy–video-assisted thoracic surgery versus muscle-sparing thoracotomy. A randomized trial. J Thorac Cardiovasc Surg 1995;109(5):997–1001 [discussion: 1001–2].

21. Biere SS, van Berge Henegouwen MI, Maas KW, et al. Minimally invasive versus open oesophagectomy for patients with oesophageal cancer: a multicentre, open-label, randomised controlled trial. Lancet 2012;379(9829):1887–92.

22. Tisdale JE, Wroblewski HA, Wall DS, et al. A randomized trial evaluating amiodarone for prevention of atrial fibrillation after pulmonary resection. Ann Thorac Surg 2009;88(3):886–93 [discussion: 894–5].

23. Tisdale JE, Wroblewski HA, Wall DS, et al. A randomized, controlled study of amiodarone for prevention of atrial fibrillation after transthoracic esophagectomy. J Thorac Cardiovasc Surg 2010; 140(1):45–51.

24. Riber LP, Christensen TD, Jensen HK, et al. Amiodarone significantly decreases atrial fibrillation in patients undergoing surgery for lung cancer. Ann Thorac Surg 2012;94(2):339–44 [discussion: 345–6].

25. Nojiri T, Yamamoto K, Maeda H, et al. A double-blind placebo-controlled study of the effects of olprinone, a specific phosphodiesterase III inhibitor, for preventing postoperative atrial fibrillation in patients undergoing pulmonary resection for lung cancer. Chest 2015;148(5):1285–92.

26. Massarweh NN, Anaya DA, Kougias P, et al. Variation and impact of multiple complications on failure to rescue after inpatient surgery. Ann Surg 2016. [Epub ahead of print].

27. Farjah F, Backhus L, Cheng A, et al. Failure to rescue and pulmonary resection for lung cancer. J Thorac Cardiovasc Surg 2015;149(5):1365–71.

28. Needleman J, Buerhaus P, Mattke S, et al. Nurse-staffing levels and the quality of care in hospitals. N Engl J Med 2002;346(22):1715–22.

29. Rosen AK, Rivard P, Zhao S, et al. Evaluating the patient safety indicators: how well do they perform on Veterans Health Administration data? Med Care 2005;43(9):873–84.

30. Silber JH, Romano PS, Rosen AK, et al. Failure-to-rescue: comparing definitions to measure quality of care. Med Care 2007;45(10):918–25.

31. Shiloach M, Frencher SK Jr, Steeger JE, et al. Toward robust information: data quality and inter-rater reliability in the American College of Surgeons National Surgical Quality Improvement Program. J Am Coll Surg 2010;210(1):6–16.

32. Magee MJ, Wright CD, McDonald D, et al. External validation of the Society of Thoracic Surgeons General Thoracic Surgery Database. Ann Thorac Surg 2013;96(5):1734–9 [discussion: 1738–9].

33. Grenda TR, Revels SL, Yin H, et al. Lung cancer resection at hospitals with high vs low mortality rates. JAMA Surg 2015;150(11):1034–40.

34. Massarweh NN, Kougias P, Wilson MA. Complications and failure to rescue after inpatient noncardiac surgery in the Veterans Affairs Health System. JAMA Surg 2016;151(12):1157–65.

35. Pradarelli JC, Healy MA, Osborne NH, et al. Variation in Medicare expenditures for treating perioperative complications: the cost of rescue. JAMA Surg 2016;151:e163340.

36. Pradarelli JC, Scally CP, Nathan H, et al. Hospital teaching status and Medicare expenditures for complex surgery: retrospective cohort study. Ann Surg 2017;265(3):502–13.

37. Mehta HB, Dimou F, Adhikari D, et al. Comparison of comorbidity scores in predicting surgical outcomes. Med Care 2016;54(2):180–7.

38. Reames BN, Birkmeyer NJ, Dimick JB, et al. Socioeconomic disparities in mortality after cancer surgery: failure to rescue. JAMA Surg 2014;149(5): 475–81.

39. Sukumar S, Roghmann F, Trinh VQ, et al. National trends in hospital-acquired preventable adverse events after major cancer surgery in the USA. BMJ Open 2013;3(6):e002843.

40. Brunelli A, Xiume F, Al Refai M, et al. Risk-adjusted morbidity, mortality and failure-to-rescue models for internal provider profiling after major lung resection. Interact Cardiovasc Thorac Surg 2006;5(2):92–6.

41. Bhamidipati CM, Stukenborg GJ, Ailawadi G, et al. Pulmonary resections performed at hospitals with thoracic surgery residency programs have superior outcomes. J Thorac Cardiovasc Surg 2013;145(1): 60–6.

42. Yasunaga H, Hashimoto H, Horiguchi H, et al. Variation in cancer surgical outcomes associated with physician and nurse staffing: a retrospective observational study using the Japanese Diagnosis Procedure Combination Database. BMC Health Serv Res 2012;12:129.

43. Friese CR, Earle CC, Silber JH, et al. Hospital characteristics, clinical severity, and outcomes for surgical oncology patients. Surgery 2010;147(5):602–9.

44. Sheetz KH, Dimick JB, Ghaferi AA. Impact of hospital characteristics on failure to rescue following major surgery. Ann Surg 2016;263(4):692–7.

45. Arlow RL, Moore DF, Chen C, et al. Outcome-volume relationships and transhiatal esophagectomy: minimizing "failure to rescue"-. Ann Surg Innov Res 2014;8(1):9.

46. Almoudaris AM, Mamidanna R, Bottle A, et al. Failure to rescue patients after reintervention in gastroesophageal cancer surgery in England. JAMA Surg 2013;148(3):272–6.

47. Gopaldas RR, Bhamidipati CM, Dao TK, et al. Impact of surgeon demographics and technique on outcomes after esophageal resections: a nationwide study. Ann Thorac Surg 2013;95(3):1064–9.

48. Brooke BS, Dominici F, Pronovost PJ, et al. Variations in surgical outcomes associated with hospital compliance with safety practices. Surgery 2012; 151(5):651–9.

49. Ghaferi AA, Birkmeyer JD, Dimick JB. Hospital volume and failure to rescue with high-risk surgery. Med Care 2011;49(12):1076–81.

50. Ghaferi AA, Birkmeyer JD, Dimick JB. Complications, failure to rescue, and mortality with major inpatient surgery in Medicare patients. Ann Surg 2009; 250(6):1029–34.

51. Pasquali SK, He X, Jacobs JP, et al. Evaluation of failure to rescue as a quality metric in pediatric heart surgery: an analysis of the STS Congenital Heart Surgery Database. Ann Thorac Surg 2012;94(2): 573–9 [discussion: 579–80].

52. Reddy HG, Shih T, Englesbe MJ, et al. Analyzing "failure to rescue": is this an opportunity for outcome improvement in cardiac surgery? Ann Thorac Surg 2013;95(6):1976–81 [discussion: 1981].

53. Birkmeyer JD, Dimick JB. Understanding and reducing variation in surgical mortality. Annu Rev Med 2009;60:405–15.

54. Dimick JB, Welch HG, Birkmeyer JD. Surgical mortality as an indicator of hospital quality: the problem with small sample size. JAMA 2004;292(7):847–51.

55. MacKenzie TA, Grunkemeier GL, Grunwald GK, et al. A primer on using shrinkage to compare inhospital mortality between centers. Ann Thorac Surg 2015;99(3):757–61.

56. Wright CD, Gaissert HA, Grab JD, et al. Predictors of prolonged length of stay after lobectomy for lung cancer: a Society of Thoracic Surgeons General Thoracic Surgery Database risk-adjustment model. Ann Thorac Surg 2008;85(6):1857–65 [discussion: 1865].

57. Aiken LH, Clarke SP, Sloane DM, et al. Hospital nurse staffing and patient mortality, nurse burnout, and job dissatisfaction. JAMA 2002;288(16):1987–93.

58. Aiken LH, Clarke SP, Cheung RB, et al. Educational levels of hospital nurses and surgical patient mortality. JAMA 2003;290(12):1617–23.

59. Ghaferi AA, Osborne NH, Birkmeyer JD, et al. Hospital characteristics associated with failure to rescue from complications after pancreatectomy. J Am Coll Surg 2010;211(3):325–30.

60. Bukur M, Singer MB, Chung R, et al. Influence of resident involvement on trauma care outcomes. Arch Surg 2012;147(9):856–62.

61. Wakeam E, Hevelone ND, Maine R, et al. Failure to rescue in safety-net hospitals: availability of hospital resources and differences in performance. JAMA Surg 2014;149(3):229–35.

62. Henneman D, van Leersum NJ, Ten Berge M, et al. Failure-to-rescue after colorectal cancer surgery and the association with three structural hospital factors. Ann Surg Oncol 2013;20(11):3370–6.

63. American Association of Colleges of Nursing. Nursing shortage fact sheet. 2014. Available at: http://www. aacn.nche.edu/media-relations/NrsgShortageFS.pdf. Accessed October 29, 2016.

64. Hillman K, Chen J, Cretikos M, et al. Introduction of the medical emergency team (MET) system: a cluster-randomised controlled trial. Lancet 2005; 365(9477):2091–7.

65. Kollef MH, Chen Y, Heard K, et al. A randomized trial of real-time automated clinical deterioration alerts sent to a rapid response team. J Hosp Med 2014; 9(7):424–9.

66. Osborne NH, Nicholas LH, Ryan AM, et al. Association of hospital participation in a quality reporting program with surgical outcomes and expenditures

for Medicare beneficiaries. JAMA 2015;313(5): 496–504.

67. Etzioni DA, Wasif N, Dueck AC, et al. Association of hospital participation in a surgical outcomes monitoring program with inpatient complications and mortality. JAMA 2015;313(5):505–11.

68. Shannon FL, Fazzalari FL, Theurer PF, et al. A method to evaluate cardiac surgery mortality: phase of care mortality analysis. Ann Thorac Surg 2012;93(1):36–43 [discussion: 43].

69. O'Connor GT, Birkmeyer JD, Dacey LJ, et al. Results of a regional study of modes of death associated with coronary artery bypass grafting. Northern New England Cardiovascular Disease Study Group. Ann Thorac Surg 1998;66: 1323–8.

70. Malenka DJ, O'Connor GT. A regional collaborative effort for CQI in cardiovascular disease. Northern New England Cardiovascular Study Group. Jt Comm J Qual Improv 1995;21:627–33.

Quality and Cost in Thoracic Surgery

Rachel L. Medbery, MD*, Seth D. Force, MD

KEYWORDS

- Thoracic surgery • Quality • Outcomes • Cost

KEY POINTS

- The value of health care is defined as health outcomes achieved per dollars spent.
- Medicare spends more than $12.1 billion and $1.3 billion per year on lung and esophageal cancer care, respectively.
- Numerous studies show the clinical, oncologic, and financial efficacy of video-assisted thoracic surgery for early-stage non–small cell lung cancer.
- Early data suggest that minimally invasive esophagectomy affords greater value than open esophagectomy in specific patient populations.
- Quality improvement pathways in thoracic surgery have been shown to decrease hospital costs and length of stay.

INTRODUCTION

In any well-run business, achieving the highest quality with the lowest cost is the ultimate goal—and the business of medicine is no different. Over the last several years, the value of medicine has been a buzzword throughout hospital administrative suites, and health care providers have felt the pressure. In 2010, Michael Porter, PhD, introduced the value equation by stating that the value of health care is defined as the health outcomes we achieve per dollars that are spent.[1] He further notions that using such a definition of value unites all stakeholders in health care—patients, providers, and payers—and if done right, all can benefit.[2]

In the realm of thoracic surgery, our aim should be no different. Surgeons must aspire to have high-quality outcomes for their patients while being cost conscientious when possible. As a result, success for our patients results in improved survival and quality of life, whereas decreased cost means more resources are available to effectively treat those who are in need. This article aims to investigate current challenges faced by thoracic surgeons with regard to achieving the greatest value for our patients.

BACKGROUND

Context: Health Care Spending in the United States

In 2014, the United States spent $3 trillion on health care, averaging approximately $9500 per person and representing approximately 17.5% of the gross domestic product.[3] Furthermore, almost one-third of all costs were associated with hospital-based care ($971.8 billion). Medicare spends more than $12.1 billion and $1.3 billion per year on lung and esophageal cancer care, respectively.[4] Moreover, data from the National Cancer Institute indicate that the cost of health care per person with either

The authors have nothing to disclose.
Section of General Thoracic Surgery, The Emory Clinic, Division of Cardiothoracic Surgery, Department of Surgery, Emory University School of Medicine, 1365 Clifton Road, Northeast, Building A, Atlanta, GA 30322, USA
* Corresponding author.
E-mail address: rmedber@emory.edu

Thorac Surg Clin 27 (2017) 267–277
http://dx.doi.org/10.1016/j.thorsurg.2017.03.006

lung or esophageal cancer exceeds $60,000 during the first year of diagnosis; and for those individuals battling cancer, costs can be overwhelming.[5] Sadly, the costs associated with dying of the disease are even higher (**Fig. 1**).

Obamacare

Over the last several years, health care costs have increased at rates faster than normal, and this is largely thought to be attributed to major coverage expansions under the Affordable Care Act.[3] In 2010, when President Obama signed the Patient Protection and Affordable Care Act (PPACA) into law, Medicaid coverage for lower-income Americans rapidly expanded. As a result, uncompensated costs decreased while hospital profit margins increased.[6] Unfortunately, despite that fact that the PPACA was designed with the goal of cutting overall health care costs, it seems to have had the opposite effect, likely because of increased access to care by those who were previously uninsured.

Current Landscape

Currently, the US health care system is largely based on a fee-for-service reimbursement system—meaning that third-party payers will reimburse hospitals and providers for all resources that are used, even if it is surrounding a complication. A recent study investigating complex abdominal surgery found that financial incentives are indeed misaligned with quality improvement.[7] A similar analysis was undertaken comparing surgical outcomes and Medicare payments after colectomy, abdominal aneurysm repair, coronary artery bypass grafting, and total hip replacement at different hospitals across the country concluded that hospitals with higher complication rates also had substantially higher Medicare payments.[8] Although the concept has not been directly proven in thoracic surgery, one must assume that similar scenarios certainly exist.

In an effort to reduce national health care spending, the Centers for Medicare and Medicaid Services (CMS) announced in 2007 that they would no longer reimburse for certain hospital complications (ie, "never events").[9,10] Five years later, in 2012, CMS further announced that they would start reducing payments to hospitals with excessive readmission rates.[11] As a result, the government's penalties have forced hospital administrators and health care providers to start focusing on improving the quality of patient care and optimizing outcomes to receive maximal reimbursement.

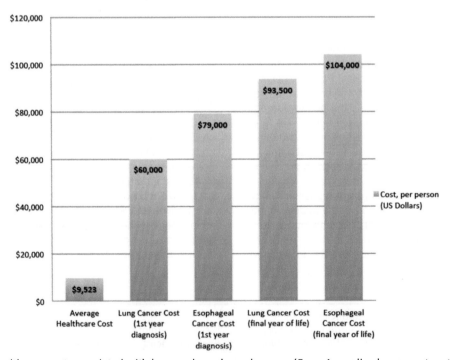

Fig. 1. Health care costs associated with lung and esophageal cancer. (*From* Annualized mean net costs of care: cancer prevalence and cost of care projections. National Cancer Institute. Available at: https://costprojections. cancer.gov/annual.costs.html. Accessed October 20, 2016.)

Implications for the Future

On the heels of establishing never events and monitoring readmission rates, the PPACA also allowed CMS to create the CMS Innovation Center. Once created, their mission was to "test innovative payment and service delivery models that have the potential to reduce Medicare, Medicaid, or Children's Health Insurance Program expenditures while preserving or enhancing the quality of care for beneficiaries."[12,13] In 2013, the first Bundled Payment pilot began. Although still in the testing phase, with multiple payment models and Diagnosis-Related Group (DRG), the concept is one that eliminates the fee-for-service reimbursement scenario and replaces it with a single payment surrounding an episode of care. Bundled payments are designed in a manner that essentially creates financial incentives for both hospitals and affiliated providers to keep costs less than the expected lump sum payment so that profit margins can be maximized.[14]

Within these bundled payment scenarios, however, it must be cautioned that patient outcomes do not falter at the expense of saving costs. Consequently, the concept of pay-for-performance is a popular idea that incentivizes providers to achieve higher-quality outcomes for their patients.[15] Unfortunately, however, there remains underlying concern that such an incentive will become non–patient centered and will have providers subconsciously avoiding complex patient care.[16] Furthermore, a study investigating early experience with pay-for-performance found that there actually may be little gained in terms of quality for the money that is spent.[17] As a result, the prefect answer still eludes us; perhaps, rather, a multidisciplinary approach between patients, providers, and payers is necessary to truly create sustainable value metrics in medicine.[18]

CURRENT DATA IN THORACIC SURGERY
Lung Cancer

Video-assisted thoracic surgery

Minimally invasive surgery has become commonplace in nearly all surgical subspecialties. Over the last 2 decades, most thoracic surgeons have adopted video-assisted thoracic surgery (VATS) as part of their practice. There is an abundance of data that show that VATS is associated with decreased pain and mortality, shorter hospital length of stay, and equivalent oncologic outcomes when compared with thoracotomy.[19–23] Because of the current health care landscape and the increased focus on health care spending, the cost of VATS has been thoroughly investigated.

In 2009, a single-institution analysis in the United Kingdom compared the costs and outcomes of 93 VATS versus 253 thoracotomies for early-stage lung cancer and concluded that operative costs for the minimally invasive approach were significantly higher; however, total hospital costs were lower than those for thoracotomy because of decreased complications and length of hospital stay.[24] A follow-up study from France in 2011 compared 98 VATS with 189 thoracotomies for non–small cell lung cancer (NSCLC).[25] Similar to their colleagues in the United Kingdom, the authors concluded that VATS was significantly less expensive, likely because of a shorter length of stay.

In 2012, an additional multi-institutional database analysis comparing 1054 VATS and 2907 open lobectomies concluded that a minimally invasive approach resulted in shorter length of stay, fewer adverse events, and significantly less hospital cost.[23] Interestingly, however, they also analyzed costs between low- and high-volume surgeons. For open lobectomy via thoracotomy, surgeon volume did not significantly impact cost (approximately $21,000 for each group). On the other hand, high-volume VATS surgeons had costs that were nearly $4000 less than their low-volume counterparts ($18,133 vs $22,050). As a result, the authors concluded that the economic impact of VATS improved as a surgeon became more experienced.

Because of concerns that outpatient costs after hospital discharge may result in higher costs for a minimally invasive approach, an additional study in 2014 investigated 90-day costs between VATS and open lobectomy for lung cancer.[26] Farjah and colleagues[26] conducted a retrospective cohort study using administrative claims data after 9962 lobectomies for lung cancer; 3069 (31%) were performed via VATS. After risk adjustment, 90-day costs were $3476 lower for VATS ($P$ = .0001). The authors note, however, that prolonged length of hospital stay likely explained the cost differences between surgical approaches; therefore, efforts to reduce cost should be aimed at reducing postoperative days in the hospital.

A recently published study took it a step beyond simple cost and outcome analysis by investigating the impact of health care utilization (costs, inpatient and outpatient visits, clinic visits, and days off work) at both 90 and 365 days after VATS versus open lung resection (**Fig. 2**).[27] Using an administrative claims database, 2611 patients undergoing either lobectomy (270 via VATS, 340 via open) or wedge resection (1332 via VATS, 340 via open) were compared. Open lobectomies had 1.28 and 1.14 times more health care utilization days than VATS within 90 and 365 days of surgery, respectively. This utilization increase was

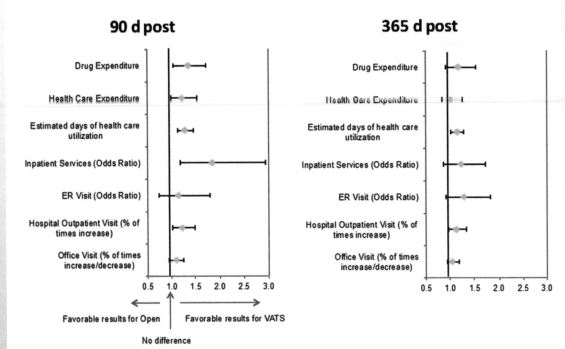

Fig. 2. Adjusted health care utilization data for VATS versus open lobectomy. Adjusted utilization data for lobectomy procedures at (*Left*) 90 days and (*Right*) 365 days. The solid vertical line indicates no difference; the solid squares indicate the mean difference, the horizontal lines represent the 95% confidence interval. ER, emergency room; OPEN, open thoracotomy. (*From* Watson TJ, Qiu J. The impact of thoracoscopic surgery on payment and health care utilization after lung resection. Ann Thorac Surg 2016;101:1278. [discussion: 1979–80]; with permission.)

associated with increased expenditures of $3260 at 90 days and $822 at 365 days for patients undergoing open procedures. Interestingly, with the exception of fewer outpatient visits within 90 days for patients undergoing open wedge resection, there were no significant differences in health care utilization between VATS and open wedge resections.

Although numerous studies showed the clinical and financial efficacy of VATS, there undoubtedly remains room for improvement. In light of impending changes in health care reimbursement, we analyzed our institutional VATS lobectomy data with regard to cost variations for the procedure itself.[28] We hypothesized that if certain variables driving cost in VATS procedures can be identified, the potential for cost savings can be improved, especially in a bundled payment environment. Clinical outcomes and hospital financial data were linked for 194 VATS lobectomies. The average cost per case was $18,637 (±$8244). Regression analysis concluded that patients with chronic obstructive pulmonary disease and coronary artery disease had costs that were $3340 and $5733 higher, respectively (*P*≤.01). Furthermore, blood transfusion, postoperative urinary tract infection and unplanned intensive care unit

admission were all associated with significantly higher costs in patients undergoing VATS lobectomy.

Although postoperative complications after VATS impacted cost variability, data showed that 39% of cost was directly from the operating room (OR) (**Fig. 3**). In a follow-up study, the breakdown of specific hospital costs associated with VATS lobectomy was analyzed.[29] The data show that highest overall percentage of costs were directly from the OR itself (**Table 1**), and most OR costs were related to OR time and stapler cartridges (**Table 2**). As a result of these studies, quality improvement initiatives to improve the value of VATS should be focused on patient risk stratification, decreasing OR time, and preventing postoperative complications.

Robotic surgery

The newest advent of minimally invasive surgery is the use of the robot. Proponents of robotic thoracic surgery argue that it is as safe and effective as VATS with comparable patient outcomes; however, the cost of the system itself, combined with maintenance fees and equipment costs for each case have caused skepticism regarding its true value.[30] A single-institution retrospective

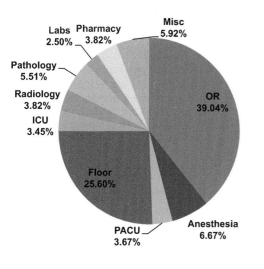

Fig. 3. Composition of hospital costs after VATS lobectomy. Based on mean costs per case. ICU, intensive care unit; PACU, postoperative anesthesia care unit. (*From* Medbery RL, Perez SD, Force SD, et al. Video-assisted thoracic surgery lobectomy cost variability: implications for a bundled payment era. Ann Thorac Surg 2014;97:1689. [discussion: 1692–3]; with permission.)

- OR
- Anesthesia
- PACU
- Floor
- ICU
- Radiology
- Pathology
- Labs
- Pharmacy
- Misc

analysis of 69 open, 57 robotic, and 58 VATS anatomic resections (either lobectomy or segmentectomy) found that VATS was not only the least expensive operative approach, but that robotic cases were significantly more expensive than both VATS and open cases (**Fig. 4**).[31] When comparing hospital length of stay and postoperative complications among the 3 groups, there were no significant differences; however, OR time was significantly higher in the robotic group. Additional analysis by the authors resulted in their conclusion that "reducing OR time by 68 minutes is required to make robotic overall cost neutral compared to VATS."[31] Further studies are needed to compare the value of VATS versus robotic thoracic surgery.

Sublobar resection versus nonsurgical options

Surgical resection is considered the standard of care for early-stage NSCLC; however, sublobar anatomic resection and nonsurgical treatment with stereotactic body radiation therapy (SBRT) are 2 options that exist for patients who are deemed too high risk for complete surgical

Table 1
Hospital costs associated with VATS lobectomy

Cost by Center[a]	Mean	SD	Median
OR	7424	1998	7012
Floor	4048	3597	3207
Miscellaneous	2020	3001	897
Pathology	1489	661	1395
Anesthesia	1258	397	1174
Pharmacy	725	1123	487
Radiology	724	542	530
PACU	692	512	522
Laboratory tests	545	776	359
Total cost	19,792	9753	17,132

Values are US dollars.

Abbreviations: PACU, postoperative anesthesia care unit; SD, standard deviation.

[a] Mean intensive care unit cost was $0.

From Khullar OV, Fernandez FG, Perez S, et al. Time is money: hospital costs associated with video-assisted thoracoscopic surgery lobectomies. Ann Thorac Surg 2016;102:943; with permission.

Table 2
Operating room costs associated with VATS lobectomy

OR Activity Category	Mean Cost	SD	Median Cost
Room rate	3908	1302	3685
Stapler	2030	860	1868
Scope equipment	399	668	343
Energy	291	300	401
Hemostasis	271	449	50
Preparation/drape	165	69	173
Drains/tubes	153	45	155
OR anesthesia activity	82	50	79
Miscellaneous	44	85	22
Wound	38	96	24
Suture	37	48	25
Dissection/retraction	5	18	0

Values are US dollars.

Abbreviation: SD, standard deviation.

From Khullar OV, Fernandez FG, Perez S, et al. Time is money: hospital costs associated with video-assisted thoracoscopic surgery lobectomies. Ann Thorac Surg 2016;102:943; with permission.

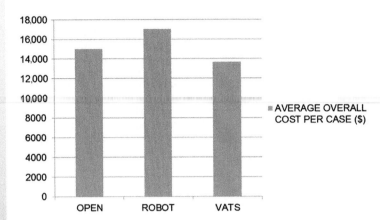

Fig. 4. Cost comparison among open, robotic and VATS anatomic resections. Overall cost per case comparison: open versus robot (*P* = .058), open versus VATS (*P* = .227), and robot versus VATS (P< 001). (From Deen SA, Wilson JL, Wilshire CL, et al. Defining the cost of care for lobectomy and segmentectomy: a comparison of open, video-assisted thoracoscopic, and robotic approaches. Ann Thorac Surg 2014;97:1005; with permission.)

lobectomy.[32,33] A recent study using propensity-matched Surveillance, Epidemiology and End Results (SEER) Medicare data compared the cost effectiveness of sublobar resection, SBRT, and lobectomy in patients ≥66 years old with localized (<5 cm) NSCLC.[34] The authors concluded that when comparing SBRT with sublobar resection, there was no significant difference in median survival (3.6 vs 4.1 years, respectively; *P* = .95), and 5-year total costs were significantly higher in the sublobar group ($77,694 vs $55,120 for SBRT, *P*<.001). On the other hand, when comparing SBRT with lobectomy, there was still no statistically significant difference in median survival (3.8 vs 4.7 years, respectively; *P* = .81), and 5-year total costs were higher in the lobectomy group ($82,641 vs $54,968). Although propensity score matching was used, it should be noted that this study is limited by the fact that patients with tumors greater than 2 cm (stage T1b or higher) are generally not candidates for sublobar resection. Nonetheless, using these data, the authors calculated incremental cost-effectiveness ratios per life-year gained and determined that lobectomy is more likely to be cost effective than sublobar resection when compared with SBRT.

An additional propensity-matched analysis, also using SEER Medicare data compared costs between sublobar resection and thermal ablation for stage I NSCLC. The matched cohort had similar baseline characteristics and overall survival, but patients undergoing ablative therapy had significantly lower treatment-related costs through the first 12 months, but the differences dissipated at the 18- and 24-month time points. Furthermore, a subgroup analysis comparing inpatient versus outpatient ablation with sublobar resection (all inpatient) found that although treatment costs are still initially cheaper, the cost differences are

much less pronounced over time for patients who have inpatient ablative therapy. Further research is needed to compare the value of surgical versus nonsurgical treatment of early-stage NSCLC.

Quality improvement pathways
Over the years, hospitals have attempted to contain costs and improve outcomes after thoracic surgery by creating patient care pathways. Two specific hospitals did so nearly 2 decades before such notions became popularized by current health care reform. In 1994, Johns Hopkins introduced clinical pathways for all anatomic lung resection patients (segmentectomy, lobectomy, and pneumonectomy) and all esophagectomy patients.[35] After pathway implementation, hospital length of stay was significantly shortened, and hospital charges were also reduced after all major thoracic surgeries. In 1996, Massachusetts General Hospital created a multidisciplinary team to standardize care after pulmonary lobectomy.[36] In doing so, the hospital was able to effectively reduce both costs and length of stay. Readmission and morality rates remain unchanged, unfortunately.

In 2014, surgeons across the state of Washington sought to analyze outcomes after lung cancer resection with the aim of creating a regional quality improvement initiative.[37] The group retrospectively analyzed a cohort of 8457 lung cancer resections from 2000 to 2011. Inpatient deaths decreased over time, but prolonged length of stay did not. Inflation-adjusted costs actually increased during the study period. Finally, when comparing costs and outcomes among specific hospitals, the variability indicates the need for standardized regionwide quality improvement initiatives to effectively increase the value of thoracic surgery for lung cancer patients (**Fig. 5**).

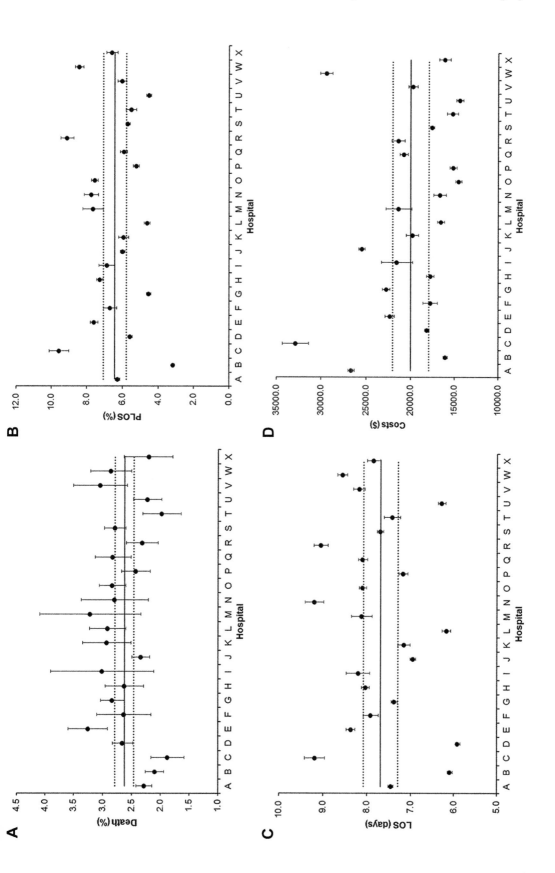

Esophageal Cancer

Transhiatal versus transthoracic esophagectomy

Surgical resection of esophageal cancer, often combined with systemic therapy, often remains a patient's only hope for cure. Unfortunately, esophagectomy, regardless of approach, continues to be associated with a relatively high morbidity rate for patients. As a result, thoracic surgeons are continuously trying to improve their technique to improve patient outcomes. A hot topic for debate is whether a transhiatal versus transthoracic approach affords better value for patients with esophageal cancer. To that end, a recent study used SEER Medicare data and propensity matching to compare outcomes and episode-based costs after transhiatal versus transthoracic esophagectomy in patients with adenocarcinoma of the lower esophagus.[38] Among 392 propensity matched pairs, there was no difference in complication rates, operative mortality, and 90-day readmission rates based on operative approach (Table 3). Hospital length of stay and initial hospitalization costs were less for the transhiatal approach. As a result, the authors conclude that transhiatal esophagectomy may confer higher value for this specific patient population.

Minimally invasive versus open esophagectomy

Beyond the debate of transhiatal versus transthoracic approach for esophagectomy exists the question about the cost effectiveness of a minimally invasive approach. A single-institution analysis compared 32 open versus 41 laparoscopic transhiatal esophagectomies for both benign and malignant disease.[39] Although selection bias is a clear weakness of the study, the authors found no significant difference in mean operating time or operative complications with the exception of intraoperative blood transfusion that was significantly higher in the open cohort. Furthermore, the minimally invasive approach was associated with a significantly shorter time to goal tube feedings, shorter hospital stay, and reduced median

direct costs. Oncologic outcomes were similar between both groups. A second study out of Canada created a decision analysis model to estimate both costs and outcomes after open and minimally invasive esophagectomy from a health care system perspective.[40] The authors concluded that minimally invasive esophagectomy cost approximately $1641 (Canadian) less than open esophagectomy and was associated with an incremental gain of 0.022 quality-adjusted life years. However, future studies are needed to confirm whether minimally invasive esophagectomy affords higher value than open esophagectomy.

Cost effectiveness of neoadjuvant treatment

For patients with locally advanced disease, neoadjuvant chemotherapy and radiation followed by surgical resection results in improved survival. However, neoadjuvant treatment is well documented to be associated with increased cost to both the patient and the payer.[41,42] Given the current health care landscape focused on increased value, a recent study sought to examine the cost effectiveness of neoadjuvant treatment in patients with esophageal squamous cell carcinoma.[43] After propensity-matched analysis, patients who underwent neoadjuvant therapy had higher mean costs ($91,460 vs $75,836) and longer survival (2.2 vs 1.8 years) with an estimated incremental costs-effectiveness ratio of $39,060 per life-year. Given these results, the authors concluded that neoadjuvant therapy for esophageal squamous cell cancer is cost effective from a payer's perspective; however, whether it is effective from a societal or health care system perspective merits further study.

Assigning stage-based value

Treatment of esophageal cancer varies widely based on disease stage at presentation, and the cost-benefit associated with different treatment modalities can be debated. A single-institution study compared the cost and benefit of esophagectomy versus nonesophagectomy based on disease stage.[44] The authors assessed medical expenses and survival time to calculate a relative

Fig. 5. Hospital-level variability in outcomes, utilization, and costs in Washington State. The letters on the x-axis represent individual hospitals. The y-axis represents outcome, utilization, or costs measures. The horizontal solid line shows the state average, and the horizontal dotted lines depict the upper and lower bounds of the 95% confidence interval for the state average. Each circle represents the reliability and risk-adjusted estimate for a given outcome, utilization, or cost measure at a specific hospital. The vertical error line associated with each circle is the 95% confidence interval for the hospital-specific estimate. The analysis is shown for (A) death, (B) prolonged length of stay (PLOS), (C) length of stay (LOS), and (D) costs. (From Farjah F, Varghese TK, Costas K, et al. Lung resection outcomes and costs in Washington State: a case for regional quality improvement. Ann Thorac Surg 2014;98:178. [discussion: 182]; with permission.)

Table 3
Perioperative clinical outcomes and costs of patients undergoing esophagectomy for esophageal cancer in propensity-matched cohort

	Transthoracic N = 392; N (%)	Transhiatal N = 392; N (%)	P Value
Median number of lymph nodes examined (IQR)	11.0 (15.0)	9.0 (10.0)	.003
Median length of hospital stay (d) (IQR)	13.0 (13.0)	11.5 (9.0)	.006
Median intensive care unit stay (d) (IQR)	7.0 (10.0)	5.0 (10.0)	.003
Hospital death	31 (7.9)	28 (7.1)	.68
Intraoperative complication	22 (5.6)	25 (6.4)	.65
Mechanical wound complication	19 (4.9)	24 (6.1)	.43
Infection	26 (6.6)	27 (6.9)	.89
Pulmonary complication	99 (25.3)	99 (25.3)	1.00
Gastrointestinal complication	37 (9.4)	49 (12.5)	.17
Cardiovascular complication	53 (13.5)	65 (16.6)	.23
Systemic complication[a]	11 (2.8)	<11 (<2.8)	.22
Reinterventions	12 (3.1)	14 (3.6)	.69
Any complication	183 (46.7)	199 (50.8)	.25
Median 90-d Medicare cost (IQR)	$45,861.5 (41,266.1)	$41,576.2 (30,598.3)	.06
Median initial hospitalization cost (IQR)	$32,533.1 (21,945.9)	$31,658.8 (15,382.5)	.03
Median remainder of 90-d cost (IQR)	$8916.33 (17,605.7)	$9365.7 (16,288.8)	.49
Discharge to home	266 (67.9)	271 (69.1)	.70
Hospital readmission 30 d after discharge[b]	44 (16.5)	50 (18.5)	.56
Hospital readmission 90 d after discharge[b]	81 (30.5)	88 (32.5)	.61

Abbreviation: IQR, interquartile range.
[a] Cells with size less than 11 were suppressed with accordance to SEER data use agreement.
[b] Out of patients discharged to home.
From Khullar OV, Jiang R, Force SD, et al. Transthoracic versus transhiatal resection for esophageal adenocarcinoma of the lower esophagus: a value-based comparison. J Surg Oncol 2015;112:521; with permission.

expense performance index; a relative expense performance index greater than 1 was defined as cost beneficial. Patients with stage I to III disease had improved survival with surgery compared to without; there was no difference for those with stage IV disease. Not surprisingly, patients undergoing esophagectomy had significantly higher medical expenses; however the relative expense performance index for surgical patients with stage I to III disease was greater than 1. These results indicate that the increased cost associated with esophagectomy was beneficial for this specific patient population.

SUMMARY

The ability to provide cost-conscientious, high-quality care for our patients remains a top priority for thoracic surgeons. Furthermore, demands from the United States government and health care administrators will hold us accountable as we strive to do so. Moving forward, future studies are necessary to delineate which procedure,

which technique, and specific timing of intervention affords the best value for our patients and their disease processes we aim to treat. Finally, while cost-containment is important, it must never be at the expense of high-quality care, as that is always our purpose.

REFERENCES

1. Porter ME. What is value in health care? N Engl J Med 2010;363:2477–81.
2. Porter ME. A strategy for health care reform–toward a value-based system. N Engl J Med 2009;361:109–12.
3. National Health Expenditures 2014 Highlights. Centers for Medicare and Medicaid Services. Available at: https://www.cms.gov/Research-Statistics-Data-and-Systems/Statistics-Trends-and-Reports/National HealthExpendData/Downloads/highlights.pdf. Accessed October 19, 2016.
4. Mariotto AB, Yabroff KR, Shao Y, et al. Projections of the cost of cancer care in the United States: 2010-2020. J Natl Cancer Inst 2011;103:117–28.

5. Annualized mean net costs of care: Cancer prevalence and cost of care projections. National Cancer Institute. Available at: https://costprojections.cancer.gov/annual.costs.html. Accessed October 20, 2016.

6. Blavin F. Association between the 2014 medicaid expansion and US hospital finances. JAMA 2016; 316:1475–83.

7. Knechtle WS, Perez SD, Medbery RL, et al. The association between hospital finances and complications after complex abdominal surgery: deficiencies in the current health care reimbursement system and implications for the future. Ann Surg 2015;262:273–9.

8. Birkmeyer JD, Gust C, Dimick JB, et al. Hospital quality and the cost of inpatient surgery in the United States. Ann Surg 2012;255:1–5.

9. Centers for Medicare and Medicaid Services (CMS), HHS. Medicare program; changes to the hospital inpatient prospective payment systems and fiscal year 2008 rates. Fed Regist 2007;72:47129–8175.

10. Rosenthal MB. Nonpayment for performance? Medicare's new reimbursement rule. N Engl J Med 2007; 357:1573–5.

11. Centers for Medicare and Medicaid Services. Hospital Readmission Reduction Program (HRPP). Available at: http://www.cms.gov. Accessed October 22, 2016.

12. Centers for Medicare and Medicaid Services. Bundled payments for care improvement initiative fact sheet. Available at: https://www.cms.gov/Newsroom/MediaReleaseDatabase/Fact-sheets/2016-Fact-sheets-items/2016-04-18.html. Accessed October 24, 2016.

13. Centers for Medicare and Medicaid Services. Bundled payments for care improvement initiative. Available at: https://innovation.cms.gov/initiatives/bundled-payments/. Accessed October 24, 2016.

14. Miller DC, Gust C, Dimick JB, et al. Large variations in Medicare payments for surgery highlight savings potential from bundled payment programs. Health Aff (Millwood) 2011;30:2107–15.

15. Epstein AM, Lee TH, Hamel MB. Paying physicians for high-quality care. N Engl J Med 2004;350: 406–10.

16. Snyder L, Neubauer RL, American College of Physicians Ethics, Professionalism and Human Rights Committee. Pay-for-performance principles that promote patient-centered care: an ethics manifesto. Ann Intern Med 2007;147:792–4.

17. Rosenthal MB, Frank RG, Li Z, et al. Early experience with pay-for-performance: from concept to practice. JAMA 2005;294:1788–93.

18. Ken Lee KH, Matthew Austin J, Pronovost PJ. Developing a measure of value in health care. Value Health 2016;19:323–5.

19. Farjah F, Wood DE, Mulligan MS, et al. Safety and efficacy of video-assisted versus conventional lung resection for lung cancer. J Thorac Cardiovasc Surg 2009;137:1415–21.

20. Flores RM, Park BJ, Dycoco J, et al. Lobectomy by video-assisted thoracic surgery (VATS) versus thoracotomy for lung cancer. J Thorac Cardiovasc Surg 2009;138:11–8.

21. Scott WJ, Allen MS, Darling G, et al. Video-assisted thoracic surgery versus open lobectomy for lung cancer: a secondary analysis of data from the American College of Surgeons Oncology Group Z0030 randomized clinical trial. J Thorac Cardiovasc Surg 2010;139:976–81 [discussion: 981–3].

22. Paul S, Altorki NK, Sheng S, et al. Thoracoscopic lobectomy is associated with lower morbidity than open lobectomy: a propensity-matched analysis from the STS database. J Thorac Cardiovasc Surg 2010;139:366–78.

23. Swanson SJ, Meyers BF, Gunnarsson CL, et al. Video-assisted thoracoscopic lobectomy is less costly and morbid than open lobectomy: a retrospective multiinstitutional database analysis. Ann Thorac Surg 2012;93:1027–32.

24. Casali G, Walker WS. Video-assisted thoracic surgery lobectomy: can we afford it? Eur J Cardiothorac Surg 2009;35:423–8.

25. Ramos R, Masuet C, Gossot D. Lobectomy for early-stage lung carcinoma: a cost analysis of full thoracoscopy versus posterolateral thoracotomy. Surg Endosc 2012;26:431–7.

26. Farjah F, Backhus LM, Varghese TK, et al. Ninety-day costs of video-assisted thoracic surgery versus open lobectomy for lung cancer. Ann Thorac Surg 2014;98:191–6.

27. Watson TJ, Qiu J. The impact of thoracoscopic surgery on payment and health care utilization after lung resection. Ann Thorac Surg 2016;101:1271–9 [discussion: 1979–80].

28. Medbery RL, Perez SD, Force SD, et al. Video-assisted thoracic surgery lobectomy cost variability: implications for a bundled payment era. Ann Thorac Surg 2014;97:1686–92 [discussion: 1692–3].

29. Khullar OV, Fernandez FG, Perez S, et al. Time is money: hospital costs associated with video-assisted thoracoscopic surgery lobectomies. Ann Thorac Surg 2016;102:940–7.

30. Park BJ. Cost concerns for robotic thoracic surgery. Ann Cardiothorac Surg 2012;1:56–8.

31. Deen SA, Wilson JL, Wilshire CL, et al. Defining the cost of care for lobectomy and segmentectomy: a comparison of open, video-assisted thoracoscopic, and robotic approaches. Ann Thorac Surg 2014; 97:1000–7.

32. Timmerman R, Paulus R, Galvin J, et al. Stereotactic body radiation therapy for inoperable early stage lung cancer. JAMA 2010;303:1070–6.

33. Schuchert MJ, Pettiford BL, Keeley S, et al. Anatomic segmentectomy in the treatment of stage I non-small cell lung cancer. Ann Thorac Surg 2007;84:926–32 [discussion: 932–3].

34. Smith BD, Jiang J, Chang JY, et al. Cost-effectiveness of stereotactic radiation, sublobar resection, and lobectomy for early non-small cell lung cancers in older adults. J Geriatr Oncol 2015;6:324–31.

35. Zehr KJ, Dawson PB, Yang SC, et al. Standardized clinical care pathways for major thoracic cases reduce hospital costs. Ann Thorac Surg 1998;66: 914–9.

36. Wright CD, Wain JC, Grillo HC, et al. Pulmonary lobectomy patient care pathway: a model to control cost and maintain quality. Ann Thorac Surg 1997; 64:299–302.

37. Farjah F, Varghese TK, Costas K, et al. Lung resection outcomes and costs in Washington State: a case for regional quality improvement. Ann Thorac Surg 2014;98:175–81 [discussion: 182].

38. Khullar OV, Jiang R, Force SD, et al. Transthoracic versus transhiatal resection for esophageal adenocarcinoma of the lower esophagus: a value-based comparison. J Surg Oncol 2015;112:517–23.

39. Ecker BL, Savulionyte GE, Datta J, et al. Laparoscopic transhiatal esophagectomy improves hospital outcomes and reduces cost: a single-institution analysis of laparoscopic-assisted and open techniques. Surg Endosc 2016;30:2535–42.

40. Lee L, Sudarshan M, Li C, et al. Cost-effectiveness of minimally invasive versus open esophagectomy for esophageal cancer. Ann Surg Oncol 2013;20: 3732–9.

41. Heise JW, Heep H, Frieling T, et al. Expense and benefit of neoadjuvant treatment in squamous cell carcinoma of the esophagus. BMC Cancer 2001;1:20.

42. Kuppusamy M, Sylvester J, Low DE. In an era of health reform: defining cost differences in current esophageal cancer management strategies and assessing the cost of complications. J Thorac Cardiovasc Surg 2011;141:16–21.

43. Lin CY, Fang HY, Feng CL, et al. Cost-effectiveness of neoadjuvant concurrent chemoradiotherapy versus esophagectomy for locally advanced esophageal squamous cell carcinoma: a population-based matched case-control study. Thorac Cancer 2016;7:288–95.

44. Hsieh CC, Chien CW. A cost and benefit study of esophagectomy for patients with esophageal cancer. J Gastrointest Surg 2009;13:1806–12.

Patient-Reported Outcomes in Thoracic Surgery

Onkar V. Khullar, MD, Felix G. Fernandez, MD, MSc*

KEYWORDS

- Patient-reported outcomes • Health-related quality of life • Outcomes research • Thoracic surgery

KEY POINTS

- Patient-reported outcomes (PROs) will be necessary for comparative effectiveness research and guideline development.
- Routine PRO data collection, along with inclusion in clinical trials and national clinical registries, is needed.
- PRO usage has been endorsed by numerous medical societies and national agencies, and has been endorsed as a possible future quality metric.

INTRODUCTION

Often in thoracic surgery, research efforts and analyses are focused on objective measurements of survival and major morbidity. There is the commonly accepted belief, particularly in regard to cancer treatment, that the best therapy provides the longest survival. Results of survival, perioperative mortality, and complication rates are objective and relatively easy to measure. However, patients undergoing major thoracic operations experience a myriad of postoperative symptoms that are not considered in these analyses and are forgotten in the concern for measuring 5-year cancer-free survival. Some are nonspecific, such as pain, fatigue, emotional distress, and anxiety. Others are specific to a disease or organ, for example, dyspnea, dysphagia, and gastrointestinal cramping. Regardless, all have some degree of subjectivity and can be patient-specific. Worries about health-related (HR) quality of life (QOL) are increasingly of greater concern to patients.

Ultimately, delivery of optimum patient-centered care (care focused on what is of greatest concern to patients) will require a greater focus on high-quality HR-QOL outcomes research (**Fig. 1**). The most accurate way to evaluate and measure these symptoms is by gathering these data directly from the patient, with no interpretation by medical providers. Such data are typically referred to as patient-reported outcomes (PROs). This article discusses the role for PRO research in thoracic surgery.

REASONS TO MEASURE PATIENT-REPORTED OUTCOMES

In the past, the subjective nature of research focused on HR-QOL has caused researchers concern regarding the validity of such studies. This is often due to methodological concerns, such as a lack of standardization in PRO measures making comparison of studies problematic, a perception of lack of sensitivity in PRO instruments to subtle changes in symptoms, and the procedural difficulties related to data measurement and administration of time-consuming surveys.[1] As a result, most studies in thoracic surgery,

Disclosures: This project was supported by grant from the American Association for Thoracic Surgery Graham Foundation Cardiothoracic Surgical Investigators Program.
Section of General Thoracic Surgery, Emory University School of Medicine, 201 Dowman Drive, Atlanta, GA 30322, USA
* Corresponding author. The Emory Clinic, 1365 Clifton Road, Northeast, Suite A2214, Atlanta, GA 30322.
E-mail address: felix.fernandez@emoryhealthcare.org

Thorac Surg Clin 27 (2017) 279–290
http://dx.doi.org/10.1016/j.thorsurg.2017.03.007

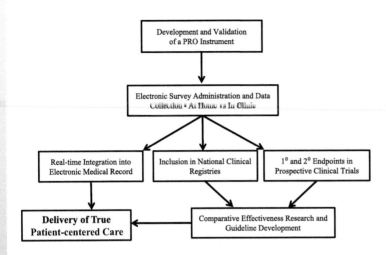

Fig. 1. Clinical integration of patient-reported outcomes research.

particularly those considered to be landmark papers, focus on more objective measures that are relatively straightforward to quantify, such as perioperative mortality, long-term survival, and rates of complications. Undoubtedly, these objective results are of vital importance because they form the basis of any treatment evaluation and, particularly in relation to oncologic care, they predominate research endeavors.

However, this approach can lead to an incomplete evaluation of treatment. Survival and complication rates alone do not provide a complete picture of the postoperative patient experience.[2] In many ways, HR-QOL measures are often of greater concern and relevance to patients, rather than minor differences in 5-year survival when comparing treatment options. Often, a patient may be willing to accept a treatment with potentially worse survival outcomes if they believe their postoperative QOL would be better. Despite this, currently, thoracic surgeons are unable to effectively counsel patients regarding the changes and differences in QOL that directly reflect a patient's experience. Further, objective measurements of survival are typically based on data gathered by the treating medical providers, who often ignore the postoperative effect on QOL. As such, the patient's voice is often lost when evaluating these life-changing therapies. In fact, prior study has confirmed that a patient's and a physician's assessments of the impact of any given treatment on postoperative QOL are drastically different.[3,4]

As greater emphasis is placed on the delivery of value-based, high-quality, patient-centered care, the importance of PROs has now become widely accepted. Patient-centered care, ultimately, is the delivery of treatment focused on what matters most to the patient. Measuring success in this

effort through objective provider-driven measures would be inadequate. PROs are increasingly viewed as the optimal measurement for the quality of patient-centered care. As a result, several major national organizations are promoting PRO research and utilization, including the Center for Medicare and Medicaid Services, National Quality Forum, National Institutes of Health (NIH), National Cancer Institute, the US Food and Drug Administration (FDA), American College of Surgeons, and European Agency for Evaluation of Medical Products, among others.[5] As further evidence of this, the Affordable Care Act resulted in the creation of the Patient-Centered Outcomes Research Institute, with the primary objective of promoting and funding clinical effectiveness research through the use of PROs.[6]

To improve the quality of patient-centered care, it will be necessary to gather PROs as part of routine, standard practice. Because PRO measures are of greater concern to patients, it is critical for prospective studies of comparative effectiveness research (CER) to include these measures when comparing treatments and outcomes and in guideline development. No longer is overall survival a sufficient metric for comparison. As a result, the FDA has recommending incorporated PRO measures as primary and secondary endpoints in clinic trials and evaluation of new drugs and devices.[7] Similarly, the Center for Medical Technology Policy has recommended that PRO measures be included in all prospective clinical CER studies in adult oncology.[8]

The remainder of this article discusses how to best gather and use PRO data, the questions and types of studies PROs can be used for, and reviews some of the HR-QOL research using PROs that has already been completed in thoracic surgery.

COLLECTION AND INTEGRATION OF PATIENT-REPORTED OUTCOMES INTO CLINICAL PRACTICE

Clearly, there is a need and an interest in PRO measurement and usage. Developing a generalizable system for clinical integration of PRO data gathering and usage for patient-centered care will necessarily require several steps (see **Fig. 1**). Routine survey administration at regular intervals would be the most efficient, accurate, and cost-effective method. The first, and in some ways, most significant step is developing a universal, standardized method for data collection that can be integrated into the existing clinical workflow and technical infrastructure, with minimal burden to the patient and the provider. This will require a robust, sensitive instrument or survey for gathering PROs, as well as a simple, efficient, and user-friendly method for survey administration.

The development of a PRO measurement instrument is a complex, deliberate process that requires multiple steps, patient and provider input, and careful validation.[5] The ideal PRO survey must be appropriate for the patient population and intervention, easy to understand and answer, sensitive to small changes in patient symptoms, and succinct enough to allow completion within 10 to 15 minutes to assure survey completion.[8] Several validated surveys and PRO questionnaires have been developed and studied in a diverse group of diseases, including those pertaining to thoracic surgery (**Box 1**). Two of the most commonly used surveys in thoracic surgical literature include the European Organization for Research and Treatment of Cancer (EORTC) Modules and the Medical Outcomes Study Short Form 36 (SF-36) because they are widely available and well-validated.

The survey must be applicable to the wide array of disease processes and organ systems treated by thoracic surgeons. Although some measurements will be universally applicable, such as physical function, pain, and fatigue, others will require greater specificity. For example, measurements regarding dysphagia and diet intake will be more applicable to the patient with esophageal cancer, whereas questions regarding postoperative dyspnea will be more useful in the patient with lung cancer or diaphragm paralysis. Thus, a single, universal survey may not be sufficient for general incorporation into a varied general thoracic surgery practice or a database such as the Society of Thoracic Surgeons (STS) General Thoracic Surgery Database (GTSD).

Khullar and colleagues[9] recently completed a prospective cohort study in which all subjects

---

Box 1
Available patient-reported outcomes questionnaires

- Patient-Reported Outcomes Measurement Information System (PROMIS)
- European Organization for Research and Treatment of Cancer (EORTC) Modules
  - Quality of Life Questionnaire Core 30 (QLQ C-30)
  - QLQ Oesophagus Module 18 (OES18)
  - QLQ Lung Cancer Module 13 (LC13)
- Medical Outcomes Study Short Form 36 (SF-36)
- MD Anderson Symptom Inventory
- Functional Assessment of Cancer Therapy (FACT) Oncologic and Organ-Specific Modules
- Gastro-Esophageal Reflux Disease HRQL Questionnaire
- Gastrointestinal Quality of Life Index
- Rotterdam Symptom Checklist
- Depression, Anxiety, and Stress Scale 21 (DASS-21)
- Dyspnea Index

---

undergoing surgery for primary lung cancer completed an HR-QOL survey at their preoperative visit, initial postoperative visit, and at the 6-month follow-up visit using the NIH-sponsored Patient-Reported Outcome Measurement Information System (PROMIS) (**Fig. 2**). PROMIS is a well-validated system of measures of PROs that include a variety of questionnaires that span multiple physical, mental, and social health domains.[1,8–12] By using a variety of short-form modules across all health domains, surveys can be customized to the patient population and disease process of interest. PROMIS questionnaires and instruments use item response theory and computer adaptive testing to adapt to the specific symptoms of a patient. Because of its versatility and advantages, it has been recommended by the Center for Medical Technology Policy as a preferred PRO measure for cancer clinical research and has been used in a variety of fields, including oncology, orthopedics, cardiothoracic surgery, transplantation, and pediatrics.[8,12]

Once an assessment tool has been selected, a method for survey administration and integration into the electronic medical records (EMRs) must be decided on. With the rapid improvement in accessibility and portability of technology, most patients will prefer an electronic survey method.

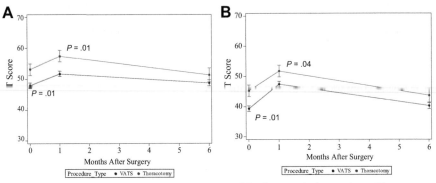

Fig. 2. PROMIS assessments of fatigue (*A*) and pain intensity (*B*) after surgical resection of lung cancer via video-assisted thoracoscopic surgery (VATS) and thoracotomy. (*Data from* Khullar OV, Rajaei MH, Force SD, et al. Pilot study to integrate patient reported outcomes after lung cancer operations into the Society of Thoracic Surgeons database. Ann Thorac Surg, in press.)

Such a survey would have multiple potential advantages. For example, a medical staff member would not be required to administer the survey and the results could potentially be directly integrated into the EMR, local institutional databases, and even national clinical registries. Additionally, electronic surveys can be adjusted and changed with relative ease. Finally, electronic surveys can be administered via a Web-based platform, as was used in Khullar and colleagues[9] study, which would be the ideal platform for survey administration. If administered through a secure, Web-based portal, such as the NIH-sponsored Assessment Center (for the PROMIS instrument) or other patient-portal, the survey can be accessed from anywhere, for example, the examination room, clinic waiting room, or even the patient's home.

Some patients, however, who are not comfortable with technology may have difficulty with such a platform and would be reluctant to complete a survey in this manner. Often, these will be older patients who are common to thoracic surgical practices. Alternate methods of survey administration would include telephone or paper survey administration. Although these methods may have higher completion rates, they require a significant labor investment with possibly added cost. Additionally, because they require manual input into electronic systems, there would be an inherent delay in data availability. In Khullar and colleagues[9] previously described study, surveys were administered electronically using handheld, tablet devices in the clinic waiting areas for most patients, with phone administration for the few of patients who missed their follow-up office visits. This system attained a completion rate of more than 90%.

Needless to say, there will be several difficulties with widespread use of PROs. For example, there

will be additional cost associated with integration into the variety of EMR systems used and development of the infrastructure needed to electronically administer the surveys. Currently, a system does not exist for most of the commonly used EMR systems.[13] These leads to the second major challenge, which will be the logistics of survey administration in both the inpatient and outpatient clinic settings. To ensure adequate patient compliance with accurate completion, PRO surveys will need to be comprehensive, yet concise, to avoid missing data. With the availability and use of smarter and more portable technology, an Internet-based delivery system would be ideally situated to meet these technological needs (**Box 2**). Other technologic needs will include the hardware necessary for administration of a Web-based survey, such as computers and/or tablet devices, and a secure server for storage of PRO survey results, such as the Assessment Center Web site, which can store results from the NIH PROMIS system.[14] Assessment Center contains a library of PROMIS tools, as described previously, thereby allowing investigators to create a study-specific Web site with PROMIS instruments of their choosing. Additionally, it allows for near real-time scoring of PROMIS tools using a T score distribution normalized to responses from the general population, which can be used to track changes in an instrument of choice with an objective score.

With the widespread use and improvement of technology, most hospitals and surgical practices now rely on EMRs. To fully integrate PRO data into clinical practice, it will be necessary to view PRO data almost as a vital sign, such as the heart rate or blood pressure, and then to make these data readily available within the EMR system in real time. This would allow the treating clinician to not only report and identify changes in PROs in their

---

Box 2
Technology needs for patient-reported outcome measurements

- Internet-based survey platform
- Electronic Medical Record (EMR)
- Hardware for survey administration and data collection
- Secure electronic system for PRO data storage, either within an EMR or off-site
- PRO integration into EMR and national registries or databases

---

documentation but also to incorporate these data into their evaluation, assessment, and treatment of the patient. For example, real-time identification of subtle changes in physical function, pain, or dysphagia could prompt further diagnostic testing or treatment interventions, such as physical therapy consults, further imaging testing, or procedural interventions, such as intercostal blocks and endoscopies. Thus, to fully embrace PROs, it will be necessary for the survey instrument to be either an integrated component of the EMR system or a free-standing electronic survey that can export normalized, interpretable PRO data directly into the EMR in real time.

PRIOR RESEARCH INTO PATIENT-REPORTED OUTCOMES AND HEALTH-RELATED QUALITY OF LIFE

Once a validated PRO measurement tool has been created and implemented, widespread collection of these data can be used for a wide spectrum of purposes ranging from large, registry-based comparisons of treatment algorithms and patient outcomes to granular use of PRO data in the individual patient to identify subtle changes in symptoms that may be a marker for a larger problem. There have been several studies that have assessed HR-QOL after a variety of thoracic surgical diseases, such as lung cancer, esophageal cancer, paraesophageal hernias, and diaphragm eventration or paralysis, to name a few.[9,15–43] Unfortunately, many of these studies had small sample sizes and used a variety of differing survey instruments (**Table 1**). Thus, they can be difficult to compare and are largely underpowered individually, limiting the studies that can be conducted and the conclusions that can be drawn. However, they do provide examples of the types of studies that can performed.

For example, 1 meta-analysis of 13 studies examining dyspnea after diaphragm plication

found that improvement in subject-reported postoperative dyspnea scores ranged from 90% to 100%.[15] Several studies have assessed symptom improvement after laparoscopic repair of hiatal hernias and fundoplications for reflux disease.[16–22] In 1 of the largest series to date to examine PROs after laparoscopic hiatal hernia repair, Castelijns, and colleagues[16] examined 85 subjects retrospectively and found low rates of subject-reported dysphagia and heartburn on long-term follow-up. In another retrospective study, Koetje and colleagues[17] compared repair with and without mesh and found significant improvements in dysphagia and HR-QOL after surgery with no difference between the groups. A meta-analysis examining the same question confirmed these results, finding no difference between repair with or without mesh.[18] Finally, in 1 of the few randomized controlled trials examining laparoscopic hernia repair that included preoperative and postoperative PROs, using the SF-36 questionnaire, Oelschlager and colleagues[19] found no difference between repair with mesh or no mesh. Multiple prospective and retrospective studies, including PROs comparing Nissen fundoplication versus partial fundoplication for reflux have shown similar improvements in reflux and QOL between the 2 procedures, with possibly less dysphagia and gas-related symptoms after partial fundoplication.[20,21] These results provide examples of the valuable insights that can be gained with PROs, which would otherwise be overlooked in studies looking at only clinical outcomes such as hernia recurrence.

Several observational oncologic studies have been completed examining HR-QOL after surgery for esophageal cancer and lung cancer, typically using the EORTC Quality of Life Questionnaire (QLQ)-Core 30 (C30), QLQ-Oesophagus module 18 (OES18), and QLQ-Lung Cancer Module 13 (LC13) questionnaires (see **Box 1**).[23,24] In fact, 1 review examining which PRO measures were used most frequently in studies of surgical treatment of esophageal cancer identified a total of 58 studies, 41 prospective and 17 retrospective.[23] Similarly, a review of HR-QOL studies after surgical treatment of lung cancer identified 22 studies published in English.[24] Unfortunately, most of these studies are limited to observational studies with sample sizes ranging from 50 to 200 subjects; however, they do reveal valuable results.

A full review of the nearly 60 published studies on esophageal cancer is beyond the scope of this article. Most studies do have similar findings, showing that there is a considerable decline in HR-QOL immediately after surgery up to 1 month, which then begin to improve toward baseline

Table 1
Summary of select HR-QOL studies in patients undergoing surgery for non-small cell lung cancer

Author, Year	Instrument Used	Number of Subjects	Time Frame Analyzed	Aim of Study	Select Findings
Li et al,[34] 2002	EORTC QLQ-C30, EORTC QLQ-LC13	51	Range 6–84 mo	Evaluate HR-QOL comparing VATS vs thoracotomy	No significant difference between the 2 groups in functioning and symptom scales
Kenny et al,[36] 2008	EORTC QLQ-C30, EORTC QLQ-LC13	173	Preoperatively to 2 y	Evaluate HR-QOL and survival in the 2 y after surgery	Half of subjects continue to experience symptoms and functional limitations 2 y after surgery Subjects with recurrence of cancer reported continued deterioration of HR-QOL, although most disease-free survivors experienced recovery
Balduyck et al,[37] 2008	EORTC QLQ-C30, EORTC QLQ-LC13	30	Preoperatively to 1 y	Evaluate HR-QOL after sleeve lobectomy and pneumonectomy	Subjects reported less impact on physical functioning, role functioning, cognitive functioning, and shoulder dysfunction after sleeve lobectomy, compared with pneumonectomy
Ferguson et al,[42] 2009	EORTC QLQ-C30, EORTC QLQ-LC13, DASS-21	124	Time from resection 2.6 ± 1.6 y	Compare HR-QOL, mood, and clinical factors in subjects < and ≥70 y	Subjects older than 70 y reported worse physical function, fatigue, and dyspnea (the differences were not statistically significant)
Sartipy,[35] 2009	SF-36	117	Preoperative to 6 mo	Compare HR-QOL in lobectomy vs pneumonectomy	Pneumonectomy had a larger impact on physical aspects of HR-QOL than lobectomy at 6 mo There was no difference in mental component scores

(continued on next page)

Table 1
(continued)

Author, Year	Instrument Used	Number of Subjects	Time Frame Analyzed	Aim of Study	Select Findings
Fagundes et al,[33] 2015	MD Anderson Symptom Inventory	60	Preoperative to 3 mo	Longitudinal PRO assessments to define symptom recovery trajectory	Fatigue, pain, shortness of breath, disturbed sleep, drowsiness severity peaked 3–5 d after surgery with recovery by 3 mo
Fernando et al,[40] 2015	SF-36, SOBQ	212	Preoperative to 2 y	Evaluate HR-QOL in high-risk subjects undergoing sublobar resection	Subjects reported worse dyspnea scores with segmentectomy (compared with wedge) and thoracotomy (compared with VATS) Poor baseline QOL scores was not associated with survival
Zhao et al,[41] 2015	SF-36	217	Postoperatively 1 mo to 1 y	Evaluate QOL following lobectomy, comparing VATS with thoracotomy	Bodily pain, energy, and physical role scores were better after VATS, compared with thoracotomy
Yun et al,[32] 2016	EORTC QLQ-C30, QLQ-LC13, HADS, PTGI	809	Single survey in 1 y survivors only	Evaluate prognostic value of QOL for predicting survival	Physical functioning, dyspnea, personal strength, and anxiety were independent predictors of survival
Khullar et al,[9] 2017	PROMIS	127	Preoperatively to 6 mo	Integrate PROs into the STS-GTSD and to describe pattern of PROs after surgery	Physical function, pain, fatigue and sleep impairment are significantly worse than preoperatively at 30 d after surgery (recovery toward baseline over 6 mo)

Abbreviations: DASS-21, Depression Anxiety Stress Scale; HADS, Hospital Anxiety and Depression Scale; PTGI, Post-Traumatic Growth Inventory; QLQ-C30, Quality of Life Questionnaire Core 30; QLQ-LC13, Quality Of Life Questionnaire Lung Cancer Module; SOBQ, San Diego Shortness of Breath Questionnaire; VATS, video-assisted thoracic surgery.
  Data from Refs.[9,32–37,40–42]

levels.[25–31] However, it is clear in these studies that symptoms can persist for several months to years after esophagectomy. For example, Lagergren and colleagues[26] administered the QLQ-C30 and QLQ–OES18 questionnaires to 90 subjects undergoing esophagectomy, finding that physical function, breathlessness, diarrhea, and reflux were significantly worse than baseline 1 month after surgery, after which they continued to improve until 6 months. However, all 4 symptoms remained significantly worse than baseline even after 3 years. In 1 of the few randomized studies of esophageal cancer including PROs, de Boer and colleagues[27] randomized nearly 200 subjects to either transhiatal or transthoracic esophagectomy and surveyed subjects at periodic intervals from baseline preoperative to 3 years postoperatively. Results of their analyses showed declines in physical function, activity, and QOL after surgery, with return to baseline within 1 year. Subjects in the transhiatal group reported fewer physical symptoms and better activity levels at 3 months. However, there were no differences identified at any time afterward.

Several studies have attempted to compare PROs after surgical therapy versus definitive chemoradiotherapy. In an observational study comparing 132 subjects undergoing chemoradiotherapy or combination treatment, including surgery in stage II or III subjects, Avery and colleagues[28] found that surgery was associated with a greater reduction in HR-QOL than chemotherapy. Perhaps not surprisingly, in a recent meta-analysis of 8 prospective, randomized trials comparing surgical and nonsurgical treatment of esophageal cancer, Best and colleagues[30] found the overall quality of evidence to be low and that only a single trial examined postoperative HR-QOL. In this single study, a significant decline in HR-QOL scores, determined using the Spitzer QOL Index, was noted in the surgical arm at 3 months after surgery. However, no difference was found between the surgical and nonsurgical arms in long-term follow-up as far as 2 years after treatment.[31]

Similarly, several PRO-based studies have been conducted on surgical treatment of lung cancer.[9,32–42] A selected number are described in **Table 1**. The findings of these studies in total describe a common decrease in physical function, dyspnea, and QOL scores after surgery. Most studies describe a return to baseline within 6 months to a year. Similar to the studies for esophageal cancer, most of these studies are either retrospective or prospective observational studies of limited sample size. However, in 1 of the few studies with a large enough sample size to perform an adjusted analysis, Yun and colleagues[32] conducted surveys of more than 800 subjects undergoing lung cancer surgery using the EORTC QLQ-C30 and QLQ–LC13 questionnaires, examining the relationship between PROs and long-term survival. After adjusting for independent demographic and clinical predictors of survival, they found QOL measures for postoperative physical function, dyspnea, personal strength, and anxiety were all independent predictors of long-term survival. In another recently published series including 60 subjects

evaluated with the MD Anderson Symptom Inventory, Fagundes and colleagues[33] administered the survey to subjects daily for the first week after surgery followed by weekly for 3 months. The investigators found fatigue, pain, shortness of breath, disturbed sleep, and drowsiness to be the postoperative symptoms to be most significantly affected. Symptom severity peaked 3 to 5 days after surgery. By 3 months, all of these symptoms had returned to preoperative levels. To date, this represents the only study to survey in-hospital subjects immediately after surgery, providing valuable information regarding the immediate postoperative impact on HR-QOL.

The study by Khullar and colleagues[9] developed a PRO survey using validated PROMIS instruments and prospectively assessed 127 subjects undergoing lung cancer surgery. These results were merged with an institutional STS-GTSD to correlate PROs with clinical data and outcomes. Subjects reported significant worsening in pain, fatigue, sleep deprivation, and physical function; at 6 months these symptoms had all returned to baseline levels. Most interestingly, subjects treated with minimally invasive thoracoscopy (n = 103), when compared with thoracotomy (n = 24), reported less pain and fatigue, along with better physical function and social functioning at the preoperative baseline assessment and 1-month postoperative assessment. At the 6-month postoperative assessment, no difference was identified (see **Table 1**).[9] Perhaps the most important finding of the study was that PRO data can be successfully linked with clinical registry data, allowing for more robust CER. Similar to these findings, results from analysis of QOL in the American College of Surgeons Oncology Group Z4032 study cohort showed significantly worse scores in regard to postoperative shortness of breath with thoracotomy.[40] Similarly, in a prospective observational study using the SF-36 questionnaire, Zhao and colleagues[41] found pain, energy, and physical role functioning all to be worse after thoracotomy.

Not surprisingly, it does seem that a greater extent of pulmonary resection, particularly pneumonectomy, can have a significantly detrimental impact on postoperative HR-QOL. Sartipy[35] performed a prospective comparison of subjects undergoing lobectomy (n = 101) versus pneumonectomy (n = 16) using the SF-36 questionnaire. Results from this analysis found a significantly greater decrease in physical function scores after pneumonectomy. Balduyck and colleagues[37] found similar results when comparing sleeve lobectomy with pneumonectomy. Physical functioning, role functioning, cognitive functioning, and shoulder dysfunction were all significantly worse than sleeve lobectomy. On the other hand, the analysis by Khullar and colleagues[9] compared video-assisted thoracoscopic surgery (VATS) sublobar resection with lobectomy and, interestingly, found no difference in any parameter after surgery, including pain, physical function, fatigue, and social functioning.

These numerous studies provide examples of studies that can be completed and valuable results that can be obtained with PROs. Unfortunately, even the prospective studies described here are limited to relatively small studies with sample sizes ranging from 50 to 200 subjects with few exceptions. This is often related to the limitations and costs associated with randomized studies and paper-based, mailed surveys. Meta-analyses attempt to solve this problem by combining data from numerous studies, particularly for oncologic studies. However, these results are limited by low-quality data, lack of granularity in regard to clinical outcome data, and difficulties with comparing PRO data due to differing surveys used. Thus, each of these studies is ultimately flawed and unable to fully answer the questions posed.

USES FOR PATIENT-REPORTED OUTCOMES

As previously discussed, PROs are the most direct measurement of patient-centered care that goes beyond simply examining survival or cancer recurrence. Once a tool for data gathering and method of implementation has been established, PROs can then be incorporated into research endeavors, as well as routine surgical practice. By measuring patient satisfaction, symptoms, and QOL directly from the patient with the previously described instruments can obtain objective measurements of outcomes of greater immediate relevance to patients. With routine measurement and use, surgeons can emphasize the delivery of quality care with a focus on what matters most to the patient: true patient-centered care (see **Fig. 1**).

For example, longitudinally collected PRO data can be used for a variety of studies, including CER and guideline development. As treatment options continue to improve and less invasive options become more widely available, comparisons will need to go beyond simply comparing survival and major morbidities. This is especially true when survival is similar. For example, PROs can be used to compare:

- Lobectomy versus sublobar resection
- Sublobar resection versus stereotactic body radiotherapy

- Transthoracic versus transhiatal versus minimally invasive esophagectomy
- VATS versus thoracotomy for a variety of thoracic procedures
- Nissen versus Toupet fundoplication, with or without mesh.

The previous research on HR-QOL has, most often, been observational studies focused on describing longitudinal patterns and variance in postoperative QOL. The few studies that do aim to perform CER using PROs typically do so in an observational manner. Inclusion of PROs as primary and secondary endpoints in prospective, randomized studies with the aim of answering questions, such as those previously described, will provide valuable direction and insights into optimal surgical treatment.

When combined with clinical data from a robust patient registry, such as the STS-GTSD, these data can be further used to compare subsets of patient populations, such as by age, gender, and risk status, and not just by treatment modality. For example, a comparison of PROs, such as postoperative dyspnea and physical function in high-risk versus low risk-patients, after treatment of lung cancer would have immense value. By using large data registries, such as the STS-GTSD or the American College of Surgeons National Quality Improvement Program, large numbers of patients can be compared using techniques such as propensity matching to compare groups and treatments when randomized studies cannot be performed. Linking PRO data to large registries would also provide the clinical data necessary to risk adjust PROs, which will be necessary for accurate CER.[43] Such results could then be used for patient counseling; prediction algorithms; and, perhaps most importantly, treatment guideline development.

There are several advantages to routine PRO collection at the individual level. Subtle changes in physical function, dysphagia, or dyspnea may be early warning signs of clinical problems. Early recognition of this through routine checks at postoperative visits can lead to early interventions, such as cardiopulmonary rehabilitation, diagnostic imaging, endoscopy, or additional physical therapy. Further, thorough prospective objective measurement of PROs will provide surgeons and patients with a roadmap for postoperative changes in QOL symptoms. This will allow for more accurate preoperative counseling for patient expectations, which is currently limited to surgeon anecdotal experience and limited data from small observational studies. Additionally, these studies would facilitate early detection of problems when patients are not following the expected postoperative course. Changes in QOL scores have already been shown to be an independent predictor of survival in patients with lung cancer.[32] Such symptoms are easily dismissed during routine clinic visits but with readily available QOL scores obtained directly from the patient as objective measures, subtle changes can more readily be identified.[44]

Given these multiple benefits, numerous national societies have endorsed the routine use of PROs as previously mentioned. The American College of Chest Physicians has gone so far as to recommend that a validated HR-QOL instrument be used to evaluate all patients with lung cancer undergoing curative-intent surgery at baseline and at follow-up visits.[45] Similarly, the FDA has endorsed the inclusion of PROs as endpoints in clinical trials.[7] CMS has endorsed the routine gathering of PROs, with future plans to possibly require them for Medicare reimbursement, as well as to include them as quality and performance measures.

SUMMARY

With increasing focus on the delivery of high-quality patient-centered care, PROs have been increasingly endorsed and recommended by numerous societies and agencies. There are numerous advantages to using PROs. Although several studies within the existing thoracic surgery literature have included PRO instruments and measures, these have been typically limited to small, observational studies. Unfortunately, at the moment, PROs are not typically included in routine patient care. Further, the lack of inclusion of PRO measurements in the STS National Database is a critical gap in current practice. PROs can be successfully integrated with an institutional STS National Database and used to gather valuable insight into the postoperative patient experience. Routine inclusion of PRO measurements in patient care will continue to allow thoracic surgeons to deliver optimal, patient-centered care.

REFERENCES

1. Garcia SF, Cella D, Clauser SB, et al. Standardizing patient-reported outcomes assessment in cancer clinical trials: a patient-reported outcomes measurement information system initiative. J Clin Oncol 2007;25(32):5106–12.
2. Birkmeyer JD, Dimick JB, Birkmeyer NJ. Measuring the quality of surgical care: structure, process, or outcomes? J Am Coll Surg 2004;198(4):626–32.
3. Detmar SB, Muller MJ, Schornagel JH, et al. Health-related quality-of-life assessments and patient-physician communication: a randomized controlled trial. JAMA 2002;288(23):3027–34.
4. Petersen MA, Larsen H, Pedersen L, et al. Assessing health-related quality of life in palliative care: comparing patient and physician assessments. Eur J Cancer 2006;42(8):1159–66.
5. Lipscomb J, Gotay CC, Snyder CF. Patient-reported outcomes in cancer: a review of recent research and policy initiatives. CA Cancer J Clin 2007;57(5):278–300.
6. Selby JV, Beal AC, Frank L. The patient-centered outcomes research institute (PCORI) national priorities for research and initial research agenda. JAMA 2012;307(15):1583–4.
7. Clinical Outcome Assessment Qualification Program. Available at: http://www.fda.gov/Drugs/Development ApprovalProcess/DrugDevelopmentToolsQualification Program/ucm284077.htm. Accessed March 11, 2016.
8. Basch E, Abernethy AP, Mullins CD, et al. Recommendations for incorporating patient-reported outcomes into clinical comparative effectiveness research in adult oncology. J Clin Oncol 2012; 30(34):4249–55.
9. Khullar OV, Rajaei MH, Force SD, et al. Pilot study to integrate patient reported outcomes after lung cancer operations into the Society of Thoracic Surgeons database. Ann Thorac Surg, in press.
10. HealthMeasures PROMIS. 2016. Available at: http:// www.healthmeasures.net/explore-measurement-systems/ promis#2. Accessed September 13, 2016.
11. Gershon RC, Rothrock N, Hanrahan R, et al. The use of PROMIS and assessment center to deliver patient-reported outcome measures in clinical research. J Appl Meas 2010;11(3):304–14.
12. Jones RS, Stukenborg GJ. Patient-reported outcomes measurement information system (PROMIS) use in surgical care: a scoping study. J Am Coll Surg 2017;224(3):245–54.e1.
13. Jensen RE, Rothrock NE, DeWitt EM, et al. The role of technical advances in the adoption and integration of patient-reported outcomes in clinical care. Med Care 2015;53(2):153–9.
14. Assessment Center. 2016. Available at: https:// www.assessmentcenter.net/Default.aspx. Accessed March 1, 2017.
15. Gazala S, Hunt I, Bedard EL. Diaphragmatic plication offers functional improvement in dyspnoea and better pulmonary function with low morbidity. Interact Cardiovasc Thorac Surg 2012;15(3):505–8.
16. Castelijns PS, Ponten JE, Van de Poll MC, et al. Subjective outcome after laparoscopic hiatal hernia repair for intrathoracic stomach. Langenbecks Arch Surg 2017;402(3):521–30.
17. Koetje JH, Oor JE, Roks DJ, et al. Equal patient satisfaction, quality of life and objective recurrence rate after laparoscopic hiatal hernia repair with and without mesh. Surg Endosc 2017. [Epub ahead of print].

18. Tam V, Winger DG, Nason KS. A systematic review and meta-analysis of mesh vs suture cruroplasty in laparoscopic large hiatal hernia repair. Am J Surg 2016;211(1):226–38.

19. Oelschlager BK, Pellegrini CA, Hunter JG, et al. Biologic prosthesis to prevent recurrence after laparoscopic paraesophageal hernia repair: long-term follow-up from a multicenter, prospective, randomized trial. J Am Coll Surg 2011;213(4):461–8.

20. Koch OO, Kaindlstorfer A, Antoniou SA, et al. Laparoscopic Nissen versus Toupet fundoplication: objective and subjective results of a prospective randomized trial. Surg Endosc 2012;26(2):413–22.

21. Broeders JA, Roks DJ, Ahmed Ali U, et al. Laparoscopic anterior 180-degree versus Nissen fundoplication for gastroesophageal reflux disease: systematic review and meta-analysis of randomized clinical trials. Ann Surg 2013;257(5):850–9.

22. Cao XF, He XT, Ji L, et al. Effects of neoadjuvant radiochemotherapy on pathological staging and prognosis for locally advanced esophageal squamous cell carcinoma. Dis Esophagus 2009;22(6):477–81.

23. Straatman J, Joosten PJ, Terwee CB, et al. Systematic review of patient-reported outcome measures in the surgical treatment of patients with esophageal cancer. Dis Esophagus 2016;29(7):760–72.

24. Poghosyan H, Sheldon LK, Leveille SG, et al. Health-related quality of life after surgical treatment in patients with non-small cell lung cancer: a systematic review. Lung Cancer 2013;81(1):11–26.

25. Derogar M, Lagergren P. Health-related quality of life among 5-year survivors of esophageal cancer surgery: a prospective population-based study. J Clin Oncol 2012;30(4):413–8.

26. Lagergren P, Avery KN, Hughes R, et al. Health-related quality of life among patients cured by surgery for esophageal cancer. Cancer 2007;110(3):686–93.

27. de Boer AG, van Lanschot JJ, van Sandick JW, et al. Quality of life after transhiatal compared with extended transthoracic resection for adenocarcinoma of the esophagus. J Clin Oncol 2004;22(20):4202–8.

28. Avery KN, Metcalfe C, Barham CP, et al. Quality of life during potentially curative treatment for locally advanced oesophageal cancer. Br J Surg 2007;94(11):1369–76.

29. Courrech Staal EF, van Sandick JW, van Tinteren H, et al. Health-related quality of life in long-term esophageal cancer survivors after potentially curative treatment. J Thorac Cardiovasc Surg 2010;140(4):777–83.

30. Best LM, Mughal M, Gurusamy KS. Non-surgical versus surgical treatment for oesophageal cancer. Cochrane Database Syst Rev 2016;(3):CD011498.

31. Bonnetain F, Bouche O, Michel P, et al. A comparative longitudinal quality of life study using the Spitzer quality of life index in a randomized multicenter phase III trial (FFCD 9102): chemoradiation followed by surgery compared with chemoradiation alone in locally advanced squamous resectable thoracic esophageal cancer. Ann Oncol 2006;17(5):827–34.

32. Yun YH, Kim YA, Sim JA, et al. Prognostic value of quality of life score in disease-free survivors of surgically-treated lung cancer. BMC Cancer 2016;16:505.

33. Fagundes CP, Shi Q, Vaporciyan AA, et al. Symptom recovery after thoracic surgery: measuring patient-reported outcomes with the MD Anderson symptom inventory. J Thorac Cardiovasc Surg 2015;150(3):613–9.e2.

34. Li WW, Lee TW, Lam SS, et al. Quality of life following lung cancer resection: video-assisted thoracic surgery vs thoracotomy. Chest 2002;122(2):584–9.

35. Sartipy U. Prospective population-based study comparing quality of life after pneumonectomy and lobectomy. Eur J Cardiothorac Surg 2009;36(6):1069–74.

36. Kenny PM, King MT, Viney RC, et al. Quality of life and survival in the 2 years after surgery for non small-cell lung cancer. J Clin Oncol 2008;26(2):233–41.

37. Balduyck B, Hendriks J, Lauwers P, et al. Quality of life after lung cancer surgery: a prospective pilot study comparing bronchial sleeve lobectomy with pneumonectomy. J Thorac Oncol 2008;3(6):604–8.

38. Ostroff JS, Krebs P, Coups EJ, et al. Health-related quality of life among early-stage, non-small cell, lung cancer survivors. Lung Cancer 2011;71(1):103–8.

39. Sarna L, Cooley ME, Brown JK, et al. Women with lung cancer: quality of life after thoracotomy: a 6-month prospective study. Cancer Nurs 2010;33(2):85–92.

40. Fernando HC, Landreneau RJ, Mandrekar SJ, et al. Analysis of longitudinal quality-of-life data in high-risk operable patients with lung cancer: results from the ACOSOG Z4032 (Alliance) multicenter randomized trial. J Thorac Cardiovasc Surg 2015;149(3):718–25 [discussion: 725–6].

41. Zhao J, Zhao Y, Qiu T, et al. Quality of life and survival after II stage nonsmall cell carcinoma surgery: video-assisted thoracic surgery versus thoracotomy lobectomy. Indian J Cancer 2015;52(Suppl 2):e130–3.

42. Ferguson MK, Parma CM, Celauro AD, et al. Quality of life and mood in older patients after major lung resection. Ann Thorac Surg 2009;87(4):1007–12 [discussion: 1012–3].

43. Bilimoria KY, Cella D, Butt Z. Current challenges in using patient-reported outcomes for surgical care

and performance measurement: everybody wants to hear from the patient, but are we ready to listen? JAMA Surg 2014;149(6):505–6.

44. Basch E, Torda P, Adams K. Standards for patient-reported outcome-based performance measures. JAMA 2013;310(2):139–40

45. Colt HG, Murgu SD, Korst RJ, et al. Follow-up and surveillance of the patient with lung cancer after curative-intent therapy: diagnosis and management of lung cancer, 3rd ed: American College of Chest Physicians evidence-based clinical practice guidelines. Chest 2013;143(5 Suppl):e437S–54S.

Database Audit in Thoracic Surgery

Mitchell J. Magee, MD, MSc

KEYWORDS

- Quality metrics • Thoracic surgery • National database • Audit

KEY POINTS

- The Society of Thoracic Surgeons General Thoracic Surgery Database (STS-GTSD), the world's largest clinical thoracic surgical database, was established in 2003 as a voluntary registry and provides participant institutions with risk-adjusted outcomes compared with national benchmarks for the purpose of quality improvement.
- An external independent annual audit of the STS-GTSD was initiated in 2010 to assess the completeness, accuracy, and quality of the data collected, to demonstrate reliability and credibility.
- In the most recent audit completed in late 2015, 25 participant sites were randomly selected, and 25 total cases randomly selected at each site, including 20 lobectomy procedures and up to 5 esophagectomies where available.
- The accuracy of the 2015 audited data as measured in 40 individual data elements, 4 categories of like variables, and overall was high, ranging from 96.3% to 99.25%, and demonstrated a continued upward trend when compared with prior years.
- The audit process is essential in validating the quality of the data and adding credibility and value to any voluntary clinical database, and additionally serves as an important tool for quality process improvement, education, and to improve patient care.

In 1989, The Society of Thoracic Surgeons (STS) created a national voluntary cardiac surgery database as a means of supporting national quality improvement efforts.[1] In 2003, a separate national voluntary clinical database was launched by the STS encompassing procedures specific to the practice of general thoracic surgery: The General Thoracic Surgery Database (GTSD).[2] All 3 components of the STS national database, including adult cardiac surgery, general thoracic surgery, and congenital heart surgery, provide participants with risk-adjusted regional and national benchmarks and provide data for research used to improve patient care processes and clinical outcomes. The database has also been used to develop predictive risk models and to support regional and national quality improvement efforts. Combined, the STS national database represents the largest repository of patients and clinical data pertaining to cardiothoracic surgery in the world.

Although administrative data are easier and less costly to collect than clinical data, administrative data has been shown to be less accurate and relevant than specialty-specific, procedure-specific, risk-adjusted clinical data as collected by the STS national database.[3–5] However, voluntary clinical databases must be proven accurate and complete before they are accepted as credible information sources. This is best achieved by external validation through an independent audit. The STS Adult Cardiac Surgery Database (ACSD) has been validated annually by an independent audit since 2006. The number of STS-ACSD sites audited increased from 3% in 2007 to 8% in 2013. As of 2015, the audit included 10% of STS-ACSD participating sites. To avoid

The author has nothing to disclose.
Southwest Cardiothoracic Surgeons, 7777 Forest Lane, Suite A-307, Dallas, TX 75230, USA
E-mail address: mitchmageemd@gmail.com

thoracic.theclinics.com

resampling, STS-ACSD participating sites were eligible for audit only every 3 years. Selected STS-ACSD variables, especially those included in risk models and outcome variables, are audited at selected sites for accuracy by comparing participant submissions with data reabstracted from original patient records in the audit process. Across all variable categories, the aggregate agreement rates for more than 100,000 data elements audited each year across multiple sites ranged from 94.5% in 2007 to 97.2% in 2012.[6]

With steady and substantial growth of participants contributing data to the GTSD since its inception in 2003, an external independent annual audit was initiated in 2010 to assess the completeness, accuracy, and quality of the data collected, thereby establishing reliability of the GTSD.

The audit process was patterned initially after the audit performed to validate the STS-ACSD, with specific parameters developed within the GTSD and audit taskforces.[7,8] An independent firm was contracted to conduct the first audit: 10 sites, approximately 5% of the 222 participating sites, randomly selected by the STS from the GTSD. Subsequent audits included more sites each year as participation in the GTSD increased and a larger proportion of participants, 10%, were randomly selected for audit. A total of 20 cases are randomly selected at each site for audit. The first 3 audits focused on lobectomy for lung cancer. Thirty-two specific individual data elements, within 7 categories of variables, were initially selected based on defined quality care measures, specific data elements essential for risk stratification within the predictive models, or variables important to the data collection processes[9] (**Box 1**). The GTSD taskforce reviews audit results annually and modifies the list of individual data elements to be included in the subsequent year audit as needed to insure the audit remains appropriate, relevant, and sufficient to achieve the stated objectives. Beginning with the fourth audit completed in 2013, the scope was broadened to include up to 5 esophagectomy procedures, in addition to 15 to 20 lobectomy procedures, audited at each site. Inclusion of esophagectomy procedures dictated that the list of individual data elements audited be modified to include variables specific to esophagectomy for cancer. Also, important and relevant changes in clinical practice, including the introduction of new technology such as positron emission tomography-computer tomography (PET-CT), endobronchial ultrasonography (EBUS), or endoscopic ultrasonography (EUS) in the staging of lung or esophageal cancer, or identification of potentially important quality metrics, such as the number of

---

Box 1
Individual data elements (32) within 7 (VII) categories comprising the 2010–2011 audits

I. Admission
   1. Admission status
   2. Surgeon National Provider Identifier
II. Preoperative risk factors
   3. Cigarette smoking
III. Procedures
   4. PFT performed
   5. PFT-FEV performed
   6. PFT-FEV predicted
   7. Zubrod score
   8. Category of disease, primary
   9. Date of surgery
   10. Operating room entry time
   11. Operating room exit time
   12. Procedure start time
   13. Procedure end time
   14. ASA classification
   15. Procedure
   16. Patient disposition
   17. Lung cancer
IV. Postoperative events
   18. Postoperative events occurred
   19. Postoperative air leak greater than 5 days
   20. Postoperative initial ventilator support greater than 48 hours
   21. Postoperative atrial arrhythmia requiring treatment
   22. Postoperative myocardial infarction
V. Discharge
   23. Discharge date
   24. Discharge status
   25. Status at 30 days
VI. Pathologic staging lung cancer
   26. Lung cancer, T (tumor)
   27. Lung cancer, N (nodes)
   28. Lung cancer, M (metastases)
VII. Quality measure
   29. Intravenous antibiotics ordered within 1 hour
   30. Cephalosporin antibiotic ordered
   31. Prophylactic antibiotic discontinuation order
   32. Deep venous thrombosis prophylactic measures

Abbreviations: ASA, American Society of Anesthesiologists; FEV, forced expiratory volume of air; PFT, pulmonary function tests.

lymph nodes removed at the time of cancer resection, prompted the addition of related variables to the list of data elements included in the audit process (**Box 2**).

Whereas 10% of participant programs are randomly selected for audit, a fixed number of cases (20) are randomly selected for audit at each site. Because procedure volume among participant centers varies widely, this could conceivably introduce bias in the analysis of some variables in aggregate. For example, 13 of the 25 sites audited had fewer than 5 esophagectomy procedures for inclusion in the audit. Also, among the 25 sites audited, the range of lobectomy procedures was 28 to 279, with 13 sites reporting 50 or fewer lobectomies and 6 sites reporting over 100. It has not been demonstrated, however, that procedural volume correlates in any way with the quality of data submitted.

A data collection questionnaire is sent to each randomly selected site to elicit information regarding the data collection process at that facility, including the facility's written process used in determining the status at 30 days after surgery variable. Audited sites are required to provide auditors documentation detailing the specific process used to verify status at 30 days, including spreadsheets used to track patients and any source documents used to verify status. Examples of source documents typically used for verification include office visits, hospitalizations, laboratory reports, or follow-up telephone calls. Operative mortality is defined by the STS for purposes of data collection and reporting as in-hospital death or death within 30 days of surgery. Obtaining accurate and complete mortality data is critical because it is the most often reported, and arguably the most significant, outcome measure. It is essential to the development and application of accurate risk models, particularly in determining observed or expected mortality, and is the metric most often used by participants for quality improvement and comparing participant programs with each other or with regional or national benchmarks, and it is essential to voluntary public reporting initiatives. To assure the highest level of accuracy when reporting operative mortality in the STS national database, the following data thresholds were recently implemented to determine eligibility for a composite outcomes score (star rating): for all cases performed on or after January 1, 2016, the operative mortality fields must have a 95% completeness rate and for cases performed on or after January 1, 2017, the operative mortality fields must have a 98% completeness rate.

A list of lobectomy and esophagectomy cases submitted by the audited sites to the GTSD are

---

Box 2
Forty individual data elements included in 2015 audit [33/37 from 2014 audit retained (1-33), 4 deleted (34-37 lined-through), and 7 additions (34-40 bold)]

1. Admission date
2. Prior cardiothoracic surgery
3. Preoperative chemotherapy, current malignancy
4. Preoperative thoracic radiation therapy
5. Diabetes
6. Diabetes control
7. Cigarette smoking
8. Pulmonary function tests performed
9. FEV1 predicted
10. Zubrod score
11. Lung cancer
12. Lung CA tumor size, T
13. Lung cancer nodes, N
14. Esophageal cancer tumor, T
15. Esophageal cancer nodes, N
16. Category of disease, primary
17. Date of surgery
18. Procedure start time
19. Procedure end time
20. ASA classification
21. Procedure
22. Patient disposition
23. Pathologic stage lung cancer, T
24. Pathologic stage lung cancer, N
25. Pathologic stage esophageal cancer, T
26. Pathologic stage esophageal cancer, N
27. Unexpected return to the operating room
28. Pneumonia
29. Status 30 days after surgery
30. Discharge status
31. Gastric outlet obstruction
32. Discharge date
33. Readmission within 30 days of discharge
34. ~~Atrial arrhythmia requiring treatment~~
35. ~~Air leak greater than five days~~
36. ~~Dilation of the esophagus~~
37. ~~Anastomosis requiring medical treatment only~~
34. **Clinical staging method, lung-EBUS**
35. **Clinical staging method, lung-PET or PET-CT**
36. **Esophageal cancer**
37. **Clinical staging method, esophageal-EUS**
38. **Lung cancer-number of nodes**
39. **Esophageal cancer, number of nodes**
40. **Initial vent support greater than 48 hours**

compared with the site-hospital operative logs, containing lobectomy or esophagectomy cases performed at those sites, to evaluate the completeness of the data. Responses to the data collection questionnaire are supplied to auditors along with the sampled medical records selected for audit by reabstraction. Audits were initially performed at each selected site; however, in subsequent years, they were completed through remote access, which proved to be equally or more efficient and much more cost-effective. The reabstraction of each data collection form is performed blindly by experienced auditors and then compared with the original abstraction alongside the sampled source medical records provided by the sites. After reabstraction, adjudication is performed of the auditors' responses and the sites' answers for all audited variables.

Mismatches are identified and agreement rates calculated for each of the individual data elements, each data category pertaining to patient status or care delivery, and an overall agreement rate for each site. Process variables are also evaluated to assess best practice for data collection and submission. Aggregate agreement rates are computed for all sites by calculation of the sum of all sites' numerators divided by the sum of all sites' denominators, for each variable, category, and overall. Each data variable is examined using the mean and standard deviation of the individual facility agreement rates. Possible relationships between data collection process variables and agreement rates are also investigated and identified. Variables with agreement rate standard deviations greater than 10% are scrutinized to identify potential contributors to high variability and associated opportunities for education or process improvement. The data collection methods used at each audited site are also examined to determine any association between data abstraction process and data quality. If a site is identified in the audit to be grossly negligent, purposely underreporting, or falling 1 to 2 standard deviations below the mean in multiple categories of data collection, the site will be required to formulate a remedial plan with the taskforce and subjected to another audit within the ensuing 2 years at the expense of the offending site. Fortunately, this has not been required thus far.

The sixth and most recent audit of the GTSD was completed in late 2015. The number of sites audited was 25, continuing an annual increase from 12 sites audited in 2012, 18 sites in 2013, and 24 sites in 2014. Twenty-five total cases were randomly selected at each site, 20 lobectomy procedures and up to 5 esophagectomies where available. A total of 20 cases were analyzed

at each site: 15 to 20 lobectomies and 0 to 5 esophagectomies. Additional lobectomy cases were analyzed at the 13 sites selected for audit that performed fewer than 5 esophagectomies in 2014, to achieve a 20-case audit total at each site. Of the 25 sites audited, 13 sites had fewer than 5 esophagectomy cases.

To assess completeness of the data submitted, a total of 1828 lobectomy or esophagectomy procedures submitted to the GTSD from all audited sites were compared with surgery logs at each audited site (range of submitted cases per site: 28–279), to determine if all eligible cases were submitted. All sites had processes in place to assure that eligible cases were submitted. Only 9 total cases from 3 sites were found in the surgery logs to have been omitted from the GTSD, with 22 out of 25 audited sites having omitted no cases. Of note, none of the cases omitted were identified as having major morbidity or mortality or other identifiable impetus for purposeful omission.

Forty individual data elements were evaluated for each case audited, with 33 out of 37 variables evaluated in 2014 retained, 4 previously audited data elements deleted, and 7 new data elements added (see **Box 2**). A total of 14,854 individual variables were abstracted and compared with submitted data elements and source documents from the medical record. The accuracy of the 2015 audited data as measured within 4 categories of like variables and overall was high, ranging from 96.3% to 99.25%, and demonstrated a continued upward trend when compared with prior years (**Table 1**).

Lower agreement rates for specific variables or increased variability in agreement rates between sites were usually due to differences in data collection processes, interpretation of selected data definitions, or findings attributable to the audit process itself. This information was provided back to each audited site during a summary conference held at the completion of each audit and in a summary report. This offered valuable site-specific information for use in education and quality process improvement. Potential problems encountered with the abstraction of clinical data include the quality of the available source material, the definitions and timing of variables captured, and the interpretation of the source materials and definitions by an abstractor.

The quality of the available source material is an important issue. At many institutions, there may be inconsistent availability and completeness of diagnostic procedure reports, operative reports, pathologic reports, and clinical records. In many cases, patients have data scattered among many charts located in different physician offices or multiple outside institutions, and the most important

Table 1
Audit agreement rates by category and overall for years 2010–2015

Year of Audit	Overall: All Categories (%)	Category: Preoperative Evaluation (%)	Category: Diagnosis and Procedures (%)	Category: Postoperative Events (%)	Category: Discharge (%)
		Agreement Rates			
2015	97.02	96.3	96.96	99.25	97.74
2014	95.01	93.54	94.25	98.61	96.97
2013	96.58	95.21	96.61	98.23	98.36
2012	93.71	—	—	—	—
2011	94.61	—	—	—	—
2010	89.79	—	—	—	—

current data may not be available to the abstractor or must be actively obtained.

The interpretation of source materials and definitions by abstractors and auditors is a critical step in the acquisition and confirmation of accurate data. This underlines the importance of providing not only clear and consistent definitions but also the need for formal abstractor training and continuing education.[10]

For the first time in 2012 and continuing annually thereafter, members of the GTSD taskforce incorporated detailed information gleaned from the 2011 STS-GTSD Audit Final Report extensively into formal written education materials provided to all database participants, as well as specific presentations prepared for the Advances in Quality and Outcomes (AQO) meeting of STS national database professionals. The annual STS-AQO: A Data Managers Meeting is a 3-day meeting for data managers, surgeons, database abstractors, and other STS database stakeholders. A major focus of the meeting is education and improving data collection. A daylong session each year is dedicated to the STS-GTSD and includes presentations on various diagnoses and associated procedures included in the STS-GTSD, recent version updates or changes, clarification of definitions of fields and individual data elements identified as confusing, and a detailed summary of the prior year STS-GTSD audit results. Variables identified as having either a low agreement rate overall or agreement rate standard deviations greater than 10% are reviewed and presented in detail with an emphasis on cause analysis and process improvement.

The audit process is time-consuming, labor-intensive, and costly. The sites selected for audit were contacted in early February 2015, and the last audit and summary report was completed in late November. The final report was received by the STS in early January 2016. The GTSD was the first STS database to pilot and verify an audit process done remotely through copies or electronic transfer of medical records from the audit sites. Prior audits were done on site, incurring substantial transportation-related expense. It was demonstrated that completing desk audits is feasible and decreases transportation costs. The cost and personnel required to complete an audit of this magnitude is a limitation but recognized as an essential requisite for maintaining any volunteer registry.

The audit of the GTSD was designed and conducted to evaluate the accuracy, consistency, and completeness of data collection and ultimately to validate the quality of the data. The high agreement rates reported for all variables analyzed in the audit process, as well as the overall high aggregate agreement rate for all audited sites in 2015 of 97.02%, demonstrate a high level of accuracy in data collection and convey that data contained in the GTSD are both complete and reliable.

The audit process is essential in validating the quality of the data and adding credibility and value to any voluntary clinical database. In addition, it serves as an important tool used in ongoing quality improvement of the data collection process, education of database participants and data managers, and ultimately to improve patient care.

REFERENCES

1. Ferguson TB, Dziuban SW, Edwards FH, et al. The STS national database: current changes and challenges for the new millennium. Ann Thorac Surg 2000;69:680–91.
2. Wright CD, Edwards FH. The Society of Thoracic Surgeons general thoracic surgery database. Ann Thorac Surg 2007;83:893–4.

3. Mack MJ, Herbert M, Prince S, et al. Does reporting of coronary artery bypass grafting from administrative databases accurately reflect actual clinical outcomes? J Thorac Cardiovasc Surg 2005;129:1309–17.

4. Torchiana DF, Meyer GS. Use of administrative data for clinical quality measurement. J Thorac Cardiovasc Surg 2005;129:1223–5.

5. Shahian DM, Silverstein T, Lovett AF, et al. Comparison of clinical and administrative data sources for hospital coronary artery bypass graft surgery report cards. Circulation 2007;115:1518–27.

6. Winkley Shroyer AL, Bakaeen F, Shahian DM, et al. The Society of Thoracic Surgeons adult cardiac surgery database: the driving force for improvement in cardiac surgery. Semin Thorac Cardiovasc Surg 2015;27:144–51.

7. Herbert MA, Prince SL, Williams JL, et al. Are unaudited records from an outcomes registry database accurate? Ann Thorac Surg 2004;77: 1960–4.

8. Welke KF, Ferguson TB, Coombs LP, et al. Validity of the Society of Thoracic Surgeons national adult cardiac surgery database. Ann Thorac Surg 2004;77: 1137–9.

9. Magee MJ, Wright CD, McDonald D, et al. External validation of the Society of Thoracic Surgeons general thoracic surgery database. Ann Thorac Surg 2013;96:1734–9.

10. Brown ML, Lenoch JR, Schaff HV. Variability in data: the Society of Thoracic Surgeons national adult cardiac surgery database. J Thorac Cardiovasc Surg 2010;140:267–73.

European Society of Thoracic Surgeons Risk Scores

Alessandro Brunelli, MD

KEYWORDS

- Quality of care • Risk models • Mortality • Lung cancer surgery • Professional accreditation

KEY POINTS

- Risk-adjusted outcome analysis is one of the main elements for monitoring and improving quality of care.
- The European Society Objective Score in-hospital mortality risk model was the first risk model developed from the European Society of Thoracic Surgeons database and applied for quality initiatives.
- The Composite Performance Score incorporates 2 risk-adjusted outcome indicators (morbidity and mortality) and 3 process indicators covering all domains of the lung cancer resection pathway of care, and it is used to verify eligibility for the European Institutional Accreditation program.
- The most recent European morbidity and mortality risk models have been developed from a population of nearly 50,000 lung resection patients registered in the European Society of Thoracic Surgeons database and are named Eurolung1 and Eurolung2.

INTRODUCTION: HISTORY AND PRINCIPLES OF THE EUROPEAN SOCIETY OF THORACIC SURGEONS DATABASE

The first version of the European Society of Thoracic Surgeons (ESTS) Database was created in 2001 as a standalone computer database (Filemaker Pro [Filemaker Inc, Santa Clara, CA]) developed by Richard Berrisford. Several units across Europe joined the project by applying via a Web page linked to the ESTS Web site and received a code enabling them to download and install the database.

Encrypted data were then exported from each unit, automatically attached to an email, and submitted to a central database. There was no fixed harvesting period, and units could submit their data any time they wished, providing more than 95% of fields were complete and valid.

At that time, more than 100 units requested the access to the database but only 27 of them from 14 different countries contributed valid data. Approximately 3500 lung resection cases were collected from 2001 through 2003, leading to the publication of the first European model of in-hospital mortality (European Society Objective Score [ESOS]).[1] The project resumed 4 years later with the creation of the first version of the online database in July 2007.

Since its inception, the online ESTS database continues to be a completely free database for all ESTS members. It was designed to include fields related to all general thoracic surgery procedures. However, lung surgery being the most representative procedure of our specialty and for the purpose of developing outcomes and process measures of quality of care, the section dedicated

Disclosure: The author has no conflicts of interest to disclose pertinent to this study.
Funding: No funding obtained for this study.
Department of Thoracic Surgery, St. James's University Hospital, Beckett Street, Leeds, LS9 7TF, UK
E-mail address: brunellialex@gmail.com

Thorac Surg Clin 27 (2017) 297–302
http://dx.doi.org/10.1016/j.thorsurg.2017.03.009

to lung cancer surgery has always been particularly detailed.

Since the launch of the first version, the online database has gone through a series of periodic (usually on a yearly basis) revisions and changes of systems with the aim to improve its quality, accessibility, user friendliness, and security according to the most recent international legislation on data protection.

In 2009, a contract was signed with Dendrite Clinical Systems LTD, Rome, Italy and most recently with Kdata, Rome, Italy to help the ESTS in professionalizing the database. This collaboration created a platform, allowing the import of data from individual units and from existing national databases. The first country to join the project was France in 2010 followed by Hungary in 2015. Following these examples, an increasing number of countries expressed their interest to join the ESTS database by exporting data from their respective national registries.

In addition to the core database, several other satellite sections have been expanded thanks to the hard work of different ESTS working groups and leading surgeons and the Database Committee (http://www.ests.org/council_committee/16/ests_database_committee).

These sections include specific fields of interest for those surgical procedures. In particular, the sections devoted to thymic tumors, mesothelioma surgery, neuroendocrine tumors, and chest wall surgery have been recently implemented.

The database is accessible online (https://ests.kdataclinical.it). A username and password are requested to login and they can be obtained by using the appropriate registration form (http://www.ests.org/collaboration/database_registration_form.aspx).

Since 2009, the Database Committee has edited database annual reports (the so-called Silver Book) from the ESTS Database to provide the membership an informative tool about thoracic surgery practice in Europe on which to benchmark their practices. The Silver Books are accessible online and free to all members (http://www.ests.org/collaboration/database_reports.aspx).

The latest version of the report included data about more than 70,000 lung resections from more than 230 units (of which, 144 contributed more than 100 cases) (http://www.ests.org/collaboration/database_contributors_list.aspx).

Data can be imputed online in the ESTS database or in case the unit has their own existing institutional database, data can be exported and submitted as an excel spreadsheet to the ESTS Database without duplicating their imputing work. Units without an internal database can use the free online ESTS Database as an institutional registry for their own purposes at the same time contributing to the European data collection. Ownership of data remains that of the contributing units that can download their own data for internal analyses.

The main objective of the ESTS database is monitoring quality of care with the ultimate purpose of standardizing and improving the outcome of general thoracic surgery across Europe. To this purpose, several risk-adjusted models and composite performance scores have been produced to be used as instruments of clinical audit.

EUROPEAN SOCIETY OBJECTIVE SCORE

The first risk model developed from the ESTS database was published in 2005.[1] The entire sample was split in a derivation (60%) and validation (40%) set. The model was first derived from a population of 1753 patients undergoing any type of lung resections (from wedges to extended pneumonectomy) for lung tumors. The in-hospital mortality rate in this derivation set was 1.9% (34 cases). Subsequently the model was validated in a set of 1166 patients (23 deaths).

The predictive model for in-hospital mortality was named the European Society Objective Score (ESOS) and included only 2 variables: age and predicted postoperative forced expiratory volume in 1 second (ppoFEV$_1$). The resulting logit equation was the following: $-5.8858 + 0.0501 \times$ age $-0.0218 \times$ ppoFEV$_1$%. When tested in the validation set, the model showed a satisfactory concordance between predicted and observed mortality, although slightly overestimating death in patients with the highest expected risk.

ESOS was subsequently applied to evaluate the performance of 3 different European units.[2] Although the units showed different unadjusted mortality rates (2.3% for unit A, 2.6% for unit B, and 4.1% for unit C) the ESOS-predicted risk-adjusted mortality rates were similar. This study emphasized the importance of using a risk-adjusting instrument when comparing outcomes between different centers or surgeons, as they may be affected by different case mixes. This report represented the first external application of the European risk model for audit purposes.

ESOS was subsequently applied by independent investigators to evaluate its predictive ability in their populations compared with other existing risk scores.[3,4] They found that in general ESOS had a better discrimination compared with Thoracoscore (the in-hospital mortality risk index based on the data collected within the French Society of Thoracic and Cardiovascular Surgery database), when applied to their patients, although it showed poor calibration in one study.[3]

COMPOSITE PERFORMANCE SCORE AND THE EUROPEAN ACCREDITATION PROCESS

Outcomes like mortality and morbidity are certainly the most widely used indicators to evaluate individual or institutional practices in this specialty. However, outcomes are only a partial measure of the overall health care quality.[5]

Inspired by the methodology proposed by the Society of Thoracic Surgeons Adult Cardiac Quality Measurement task force,[6] the ESTS database committee developed a Composite Performance Score (CPS) for lung surgery.[7]

The method consisted of developing standardized outcome and process indicators covering all temporal domains (preoperative, intraoperative, and postoperative) of the index operation—lung cancer surgery. All the selected process indicators were evidence based according to existing guidelines.

The initial CPS was developed from the first version of the ESTS database including approximately 1600 patients undergoing lung cancer surgery.[7] Two processes (proportion of patients with low predicted postoperative FEV_1 with diffusing capacity of the lungs for carbon monoxide measured before surgery and the proportion of patients receiving a systematic lymph node dissection during the operation) and 2 outcome indicators (risk-adjusted morbidity and mortality) were selected at that time. Each of these indicators were rescaled according to their cumulative standard deviations to obtain individual standardized indicators, which were in turn summed to obtain a composite score of each contributing thoracic surgery unit. Ten units were ranked either by using their risk-adjusted mortality or their CPS. By using the CPS, all 10 units tested in the original study changed their position compared with the rank obtained by using the mortality alone. Four of them moved more than one place in the rating scale.

The initial morbidity and mortality models were periodically refined in subsequent analyses on increasingly larger populations registered in the ESTS database. A more recent study published from the ESTS Database Committee updated the outcome models, changed one of the process indicators (by removing the criteria of low FEV_1 to expect measurement of diffusing capacity of the lungs for carbon monoxidebefore the operation), and included in the CPS a third process indicator (the proportion of patients with clinical N2 undergoing preoperative invasive mediastinal staging).

The latter analysis was based on more than 4000 patients registered in the online version of the ESTS database from 2007 to 2010 (a different population compared with that of the original publication).

The outcome models derived in this latter study were as follows:

Mortality logit: $-3.22 + 1.049 \times$ pneumonectomy (coded as 1 vs 0 lobectomy) $+ 0.928 \times$ cardiac comorbidity (coded as 1 and including coronary artery disease [CAD], any previous cardiac surgery, history and treatment of arrhythmia, congestive heart failure, hypertension) $-0.0175 \times$ ppoFEV$_1$%

Cardiopulmonary morbidity logit: $-3.52 + 0.659 \times$ pneumonectomy $+ 0.403 \times$ extended resection (coded as 1 and including chest wall resection, pleuropneumonectomy, completion operation, intrapericardial operation) $+ 0.322 \times$ cardiac comorbidity $-0.0065 \times$ ppoFEV$_1$% $+ 0.0315 \times$ age.

The CPS is currently the main factor determining eligibility of centers for the ESTS Institutional Accreditation Program, which was launched in 2011 (http://www.ests.org/collaboration/ests_quality_certification_programme.aspx). In addition to the database participation and a positive CPS (score >0), units must meet certain structural, procedural, and qualification criteria according to the European guidelines on structure and qualification of general thoracic surgery.[8] Eligible units are invited to apply for the program and accept a local inspection by an external auditing team, made up of representatives from the data auditing company and a thoracic surgeon selected by the Database Committee.

The audit focuses on a random sample of data submitted to the ESTS Database to verify their quality and correspondence with source data file and on the structural/procedural and qualification characteristics of the unit. The auditors will then produce a report to be reviewed by the Database Committee and ESTS Executive Committee, which will deliberate on the institutional accreditation of that unit.

The accreditation currently represents only a quality label, aimed at improving standards of quality of care in our specialty across Europe.

EUROLUNG

As mentioned above, the previous outcome models were developed from populations of few thousands of lung resection patients. During the following years, the ESTS Database has continued to grow and includes currently more than 50,000 anatomic lung resections. It seemed appropriate to update the old risk models with more reliable ones to increase their representativeness and generalizability. Therefore, the ESTS Database Committee recently published new cardiopulmonary and mortality models called *Eurolung1* and *Eurolung2*, respectively and based on 47,960 anatomic lung resections registered in the ESTS database from July 2007 to August 2015.[9] Thirteen percent of patients were operated on by video-assisted thoracoscopic surgery. Cardiopulmonary morbidity and 30-day mortality rates were 18.4% and 2.7%, respectively. Mortality rate was 6.8% after pneumonectomy, 2.3% after lobectomy/bilobectomy, and 1.4% after segmentectomy. Two types of models were generated for each outcome: a logistic regression equation and an aggregate score (more user friendly). The variables were firsts elected by univariable analysis and then entered in a stepwise logistic regression analysis, finally validated by bootstrap resampling technique.

The following logistic cardiopulmonary morbidity model was developed (*Logistic EuroLung1*): logit (morbidity) = $-2.465 + 0.497 \times$ sex male (coded 1 for male and 0 for female) $+ 0.026 \times$ age $+ 0.231 \times$ CAD (coded 1 for presence of CAD) $+ 0.371 \times$ cerebrovascular disease (CVD; coded 1 for presence of CVD) $+ 0.152 \times$ chronic kidney disease (coded 1 for presence of chronic kidney disease) $- 0.015 \times$ ppoFEV$_1$ $+ 0.514X$ extended resections (coded 1 for presence of extended resection) $+ 0.497 \times$ thoracotomy (coded 1 for thoracotomy and 0 for video-assisted thoracoscopic surgery). When the morbidity predicted by Eurolung1 was plotted against the observed one, the 2 lines were almost superimposed, indicating high precision of the

model (**Fig. 1**). The aggregate score was developed by assigning proportionally weighted points to the regression coefficients (1 point to the smallest coefficient): chronic kidney disease, 1 point; CAD and CVD2, 2 points; age greater than 65, sex male, thoracotomy, extended resections and ppoFEV$_1$ less than 70%, 3 points. Individual scores varied from 0 to 19 points. Patients with scores associated with similar risk of morbidity were then grouped into 6 classes of incremental morbidity risk ($P<.0001$) (**Table 1**).

Similarly, a 30-day mortality regression model was developed. The following logistic mortality model was generated (Logistic EuroLung2): logit (mortality) = $-5.82 + 0.903 \times$ sex male (coded 1 for male and 0 for female) $+ 0.044 \times$

Table 1
Distribution of complications according to the Eurolung1 aggregate morbidity score

Eurolung 1 Score	Morbidity Rate (%)
0–1	5.2
2–4	8.2
5–7	14.3
8–11	21.6
12–16	32.4
17–19	43.1

Data from Brunelli A, Salati M, Rocco G, et al. European risk models for morbidity (EuroLung1) and mortality (EuroLung2) to predict outcome following anatomic lung resections: an analysis from the European Society of Thoracic Surgeons database. Eur J Cardiothorac Surg 2016;51(3):490–7.

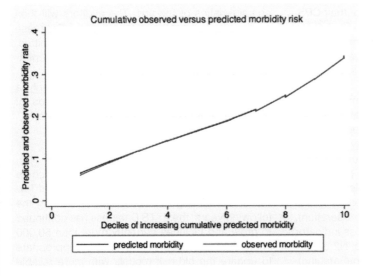

Cumulative observed versus predicted morbidity risk

Fig. 1. Plots of the predicted and observed cardiopulmonary morbidity rates with the patients ordered by increasing risk of cardiopulmonary morbidity according to Eurolung1. (*From* Brunelli A, Salati M, Rocco G, et al. European risk models for morbidity (EuroLung1) and mortality (EuroLung2) to predict outcome following anatomic lung resections: an analysis from the European Society of Thoracic Surgeons database. Eur J Cardiothorac Surg 2016;51(3):493; with permission.)

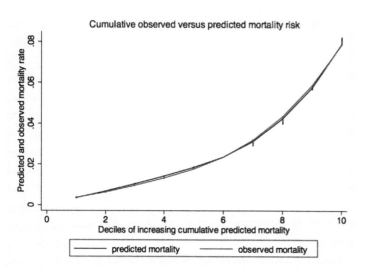

Fig. 2. Plots of the predicted and observed mortality rates with the patients ordered by increasing risk of mortality according to Euro-lung2. (*From* Brunelli A, Salati M, Rocco G, et al. European risk models for morbidity (EuroLung1) and mortality (EuroLung2) to predict outcome following anatomic lung resections: an analysis from the European Society of Thoracic Surgeons database. Eur J Cardiothorac Surg 2016;51(3):493; with permission.)

age + 0.264 × CAD (coded 1 for presence of CAD) + 0.582 × CVD (coded 1 for presence of CVD) −0.064 × body mass index + 0.300 × extended resection (coded 1 for extended resection) + 0.929X pneumonectomy (coded 1 for pneumonectomy and 0 for lesser resection) + 0.894 × thoracotomy (coded 1 for thoracotomy and 0 for video-assisted thoracoscopic surgery) – 0.009 × ppoFEV$_1$. When the mortality predicted by Eurolung2 was plotted against the observed one, the 2 lines were again almost superimposed, indicating high precision of the mortality model (**Fig. 2**). In comparison, the old ESOS model published in 2005 showed a consistent underestimation of mortality when plotted in the current set of patients (**Fig. 3**).

Using the similar methodology described for the aggregate morbidity model, an aggregate risk score was developed also for mortality (Aggregate EuroLung2): ppoFEV$_1$ less than 70%, CAD and extended resections, 1 point; age greater than 65 and CVD, 2 points; sex, thoracotomy, body mass index less than 18.5 and pneumonectomy, 3 points. The total scores varied from 0 to 17 points, and patients with scores associated with similar risk of mortality were grouped in 6 classes of incremental risk of mortality (*P*<.0001) (**Table 2**). The new models of morbidity and mortality have been recently incorporated in the CPS to replace the outdated versions.

The models in the form of aggregate scores represent a simpler instrument of risk assessment,

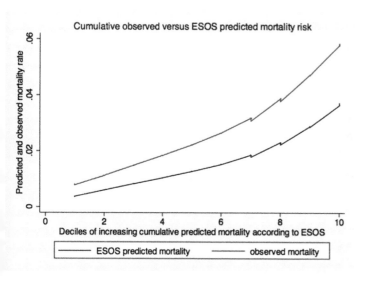

Fig. 3. Plots of the predicted and observed mortality rates with the patients ordered by increasing risk of mortality according to ESOS when applied to the current population of lung resection patients in the ESTS database.

Table 2
Distribution of mortality according to the Eurolung2 aggregate morbidity score

Eurolung 2 Score	Mortality Rate (%)
0–3	0.4
4–6	1.4
7–8	2.9
9–11	5.2
12–14	11.3
15–17	29.4

Data from Brunelli A, Salati M, Rocco G, et al. European risk models for morbidity (EuroLung1) and mortality (EuroLung2) to predict outcome following anatomic lung resections: an analysis from the European Society of Thoracic Surgeons database. Eur J Cardiothorac Surg 2016;51(3):490–7.

which can assist the clinicians during the preoperative counseling phase. In fact, they can be used as information aid tools to more accurately inform the physician-patient shared decision-making process.

SUMMARY

Risk-adjusted outcome analysis is pivotal for monitoring and improving surgical performance and quality of care, which is one of the missions of ESTS. The society has established an online database more than 15 years ago, which is continuously expanding, allowing for the creation of more accurate and reliable risk models. We have herein summarized the several risk models generated during the last years of activity of the database and that have been used for ESTS quality initiatives.

REFERENCES

1. Berrisford R, Brunelli A, Rocco G, et al. The European Thoracic Surgery Database project: modelling the risk of in-hospital death following lung resection. Eur J Cardiothorac Surg 2005;28:306–11.
2. Brunelli A, Varela G, Van Schil P, et al. Multicentric analysis of performance after major lung resections by using the European Society Objective Score (ESOS). Eur J Cardiothorac Surg 2008;33:284–8.
3. Poullis M, McShane J, Shaw M, et al. Prediction of in-hospital mortality following pulmonary resections: improving on current risk models. Eur J Cardiothorac Surg 2013;44(2):238–42.
4. Barua A, Handagala SD, Socci L, et al. Accuracy of two scoring systems for risk stratification in thoracic surgery. Interact Cardiovasc Thorac Surg 2012;14(5):556–9.
5. Brunelli A, Rocco G. Clinical and nonclinical indicators of performance in thoracic surgery. Thorac Surg Clin 2007;17:369–77.
6. Shahian DM, Edwards FH, Ferraris VA, et al. Report of the STS Quality Measurement Task Force. Quality measurement in adult cardiac surgery: part 1-Conceptual framework and measure selection. Ann Thorac Surg 2007;83:S3–12.
7. Brunelli A, Berrisford RG, Rocco G, et al. The European Thoracic Database project: Composite Performance Score to measure quality of care major lung resection. Eur J Cardiothorac Surg 2009;35:769–77.
8. Brunelli A, Falcoz PE, D'Amico T, et al. European guidelines on structure and qualification of general thoracic surgery. Eur J Cardiothorac Surg 2014; 45(5):779–86.
9. Brunelli A, Salati M, Rocco G, et al. European risk models for morbidity (EuroLung1) and mortality (EuroLung2) to predict outcome following anatomic lung resections: an analysis from the European Society of Thoracic Surgeons database. Eur J Cardiothorac Surg 2016;51(3):490–7.

International General Thoracic Surgery Database Collaboration

Christopher W. Seder, MD[a],*,
Pierre-Emmanuel Falcoz, MD, PhD[b], Michele Salati, MD[c]

KEYWORDS

- Database • Outcomes • General thoracic surgery

KEY POINTS

- One of the recent goals of the Society of Thoracic Surgeons General Thoracic Surgery Database (STS GTSD) Task Force has been an increased focus on international database collaboration.
- To date, such collaboration has primarily been with the European Society of Thoracic Surgeons (ESTS) Registry Task Force.
- Collaboration with other international databases remains an interest of the STS GTSD and ESTS registry Task Forces.

INTRODUCTION

Over the past decade, large clinical databases have been increasingly used for benchmarking, quality improvement, and the identification of factors associated with morbidity and mortality. The Society of Thoracic Surgeons General Thoracic Surgery Database (STS GTSD) is the world's largest clinical general thoracic surgery database.[1] One of the recent goals of the STS GTSD Task Force has been an increased focus on international database collaboration. To date, such collaboration has primarily been with the European Society of Thoracic Surgeons (ESTS) Registry Task Force. This collaboration was initiated in 2012, and was in large part due to the initial efforts of Dr Cameron Wright, the chair of the STS GTSD Task Force, and Dr Alessandro Brunelli, the Director of the ESTS Registry Task Force, at the time (**Fig. 1**). A joint STS-ESTS database Task Force meeting is held annually, during which, brainstorming and planning takes place for current and future projects. This article provides an overview of the STS GTSD and ESTS registry, recent collaborative projects, obstacles encountered, and future directions for the databases.

THE SOCIETY OF THORACIC SURGEONS GENERAL THORACIC SURGERY DATABASE

Established in 2002, the STS GTSD is an audited, voluntary database that provides participants with risk-adjusted twice-yearly performance reports comparing institutional outcomes against national data. Participation in the STS GTSD has increased each year since its inception, with 209 participants contributing to the spring 2016 data harvest. As of September 2, 2016, the STS GTSD included data from 912 surgeons (885 thoracic surgeons, 26 general surgeons, and 1 pulmonologist) at 283 US and Canadian institutions for a total of 459,097 operations. In addition, 6 surgeons in the United Arab Emirates and 2 surgeons in Singapore contribute to the database. **Table 1** summarizes the STS GTSD aggregate outcomes for lobectomy, pneumonectomy, and esophagectomy (2012–2014,

[a] Department of Cardiovascular and Thoracic Surgery, Rush University Medical Center, 1725 West Harrison Street, Suite 774, Chicago, IL 60612, USA; [b] Department of Thoracic Surgery, Nouvel Hopital Civil, 1 Place de l'hopital, Strasbourg 67091, France; [c] Unit of Thoracic Surgery, AOU Ospedali Riuniti - Ancona, Italy, Via Conca 71, Ancona 60126, Italy
* Corresponding author.
E-mail address: christopher_w_seder@rush.edu

Thorac Surg Clin 27 (2017) 303–313
http://dx.doi.org/10.1016/j.thorsurg.2017.03.010
1547-4127/17/© 2017 Elsevier Inc. All rights reserved.

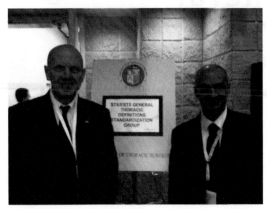

Fig. 1. Drs Cameron Wright and Alessandro Brunelli at the joint STS-ESTS general thoracic definitions standardization meeting in 2012.

lobectomy and pneumonectomy; 2011–2014, esophagectomy).[2]

The STS GTSD Task Force is a voluntary committee that provides oversight of the database. All data are entered locally by clinical database managers or surgeons and uploaded twice-yearly to Duke Clinical Research Institute, which serves as the data warehouse and analysis center for the STS National Database. The content of the database is reviewed by the GTSD Task Force and updates are made every 3 years. This process attempts to optimize data collection for recent advances in in general thoracic surgery, while ensuring that the utility of the data previously entered is maintained.

Since 2010, annual STS GTSD audits have been performed.[3] These have demonstrated high agreement rates with hospital records, validating the accuracy and completeness of the STS GTSD. In 2012, several quality measures derived from the STS GTSD were endorsed by the National Quality Forum, with ongoing efforts for endorsement of additional measures.[4]

Every year, the STS GTSD Task Force undertakes multiple projects using the database. In 2015, the STS risk models for lung resection and esophagectomy for cancer were updated, facilitating the reporting of modern observed:expected morbidity and mortality ratios for participating institutions.[5,6] Similarly, composite quality measures for lobectomy for lung cancer[7] and esophagectomy for esophageal cancer[8] were developed, allowing the designation of participating institutions as 1-star, 2-star, or 3-star programs based on their risk-adjusted outcomes. The STS GTSD Task Force is currently in the process of developing a public reporting Web site, where patients can go to compare outcomes of participating institutions. Finally, international collaboration with the ESTS registry remains a focus of the STS GTSD, with multiple collaborative projects having been recently completed, with more on the horizon.

EUROPEAN SOCIETY OF THORACIC SURGERY DATABASE

The ESTS registry is an international, voluntary database endorsed and managed by the European Society of Thoracic Surgery. This registry is designed as a modular database, in which information flows are simple and repetitive and data are imputed by using an online platform (https://ests.kdataclinical.it).

The original dataset has changed over time. At present, it consists of 5 elements: the central database, which houses clinical data on patients who underwent lung resection, and 4 other satellite modules (thymic module, mesothelioma module, neuroendocrine tumors module, and chest wall module) that, maintaining the same coding system and the same language of the principal repository, were developed to collect pertinent data for each respective surgical procedure. A growing number of procedures have been captured in the ESTS registry since its foundation in 2007, with 10,000 to 15,000 new cases collected annually (**Fig. 2**). It houses data from 170 European active contributors (submitting at least 100 procedures each) and

Table 1			
The Society of Thoracic Surgeons General Thoracic Surgery Database aggregate outcomes (2012–2014, lobectomy and pneumonectomy; 2011–2014, esophagectomy)			
Procedure	Major Morbidity, %	30-d Mortality, %	LOS, d[a] Median (IQR)
Lobectomy[5]	9.4	1.3	4 (4)
Pneumonectomy[5]	16	5	5 (4)
Esophagectomy[6]	33.1	3.4	10 (7)

Abbreviations: IQR, interquartile range; LOS, length of stay.
[a] Data from 21st Data Analysis of the Society of Thoracic Surgeons General Thoracic Surgery Database.
From Seder CW, Wright CD, Chang AC, et al. The Society of Thoracic Surgeons General Thoracic Surgery Database update on outcomes and quality. Ann Thorac Surg 2016;101(5):1646–54.

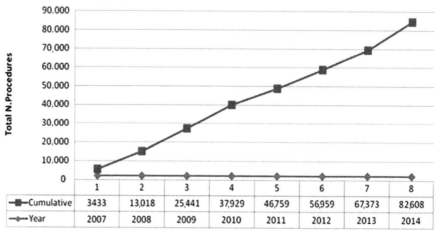

	1	2	3	4	5	6	7	8
■ Cumulative	3433	13,018	25,441	37,929	46,759	56,959	67,373	82,608
♦ Year	2007	2008	2009	2010	2011	2012	2013	2014

Fig. 2. Cumulative total procedures collected in the ESTS Registry (2007–2014).

15 non-European active contributors. Currently, the ESTS registry reposits data for thoracic surgery units in 24 different countries.

The ESTS registry collects data from European and non-European thoracic surgery units, where at least 1 staff surgeon, who is a member of the ESTS, is allowed to access the online platform using a unique identifier obtained by formal request. The records are uploaded anonymously and data are stored and managed by an external company (K-Data Clinical, Rome, Italy), which operates in full compliance with existing international data protection legislation. Apart from the prospectively collected data from single institutions, the system is able to receive intermittent (usually annually) large data uploads from national registries, after formal agreement and technical validation of the data-capturing activities. This form of contribution is currently in place for the French and the Hungarian national registries. All the contributors to the ESTS registry have the rights to their own data for clinical, administrative, and scientific purposes. Moreover, the participants can propose specific research projects to the ESTS Database Task Force to access data derived from the entire database: http://www.ests.org/collaboration/ests_database_rules_for_publications_and_presentations.aspx.

The main purposes of the ESTS Database are to improve quality of care and education in European thoracic surgery. Since 2005, data stored within this registry have been used for 3 different purposes. First, risk models for performing lung resections in Europe have been developed with ESTS registry data.[9,10] Second, the ESTS Database Committee published studies with the aim of estimating and increasing the quality of care using the ESTS contributors as platform for analysis. A multiparametric performance indicator (Composite Performance Score [CPS]) was developed and used for assessing the outcomes for different aspects of clinical practice.[11,12] The CPS is currently one of the most important parameters evaluated for obtaining the institutional clinical accreditation by the ESTS (http://www.ests.org/collaboration/ests_quality_certification_programme.aspx). Third, the ESTS Database has been used to perform specific data quality studies to develop methodologies for assessing the quality of the registry, as well as the quality of data submitted by each unit contributing to the database.[13,14]

INTERNATIONAL DATABASE COLLABORATION

International collaboration with the ESTS has been a focus of the STS GTSD Task Force in the past number of years. Recent endeavors have included harmonization of terminology between the 2 databases and performing an intersocietal comparison of pulmonary resection practices and short-term outcomes.[15,16]

The STS GTSD and ESTS registry were independently created to objectively measure and report processes and outcomes for quality improvement purposes. However, early attempts at comparison of the databases were limited by variation in the information collected and data definitions. To address this, members of the STS GTSD and ESTS Database Task Forces worked to harmonize definitions, resulting in standardization between the databases. Specifically, members of the STS GTSD and ESTS Database Task Forces identified a list of more than 60 variables of common interest. This included 50 variables present in both registries and 12 present in at least one of the registries **(Tables 2 and 3).** For each variable,

Table 2
A list of all variables with agreed-on definitions in the Society of Thoracic Surgeons General Thoracic Surgery Database and the European Society of Thoracic Surgeons database

	Variable	Definition
1	Date of birth	Patient's date of birth using 4-digit format for year (dd/mm/yyyy)
2	Age	Patient's age in years, at time of operation; this should be calculated from the date of birth and the date of operation
3	Gender	Patient's gender at birth as either male or female
4	Height, m	Height of the patient in meters at the time of operation
5	Weight, kg	Weight of the patient in kilograms at the time of operation
6	Current treatment for hypertension	Patient has a diagnosis of hypertension, documented by current pharmacologic therapy, diet, and/or exercise to control hypertension
7	Current treatment for cardiac failure	Patient is currently using pharmacologic therapy to treat congestive heart failure; heart failure is defined as physician documentation or report of any of the following clinical symptoms of heart failure described as unusual dyspnea on light exertion, recurrent dyspnea occurring in the supine position, fluid retention; or the description of rales, jugular venous distention, pulmonary edema on physical examination, or pulmonary edema on chest roentgenogram; a low ejection fraction without clinical evidence of heart failure does not qualify as heart failure
8	Coronary artery disease	Patient has a history of coronary artery disease (CAD) as evidenced by 1 of the following: 1. Currently receiving medical treatment for CAD 2. History of myocardial infarction 3. Prior CV intervention including, but not limited to, CABG, PCI, or both
9	Any previous cardiac surgical procedures	Patient has undergone any prior cardiac surgical procedure that required a general anesthetic and an incision into the mediastinum or chest
10	Neoadjuvant chemotherapy	Patient received preoperative chemotherapy (or chemoradiotherapy) for the current thoracic malignancy; do not report treatment for prior cancers
11	Neoadjuvant radiotherapy	Patient received preoperative radiotherapy (or chemoradiotherapy) for the current thoracic malignancy; do not report treatment for prior cancers
12	Other comorbidities: CVA	Patient has a history of cerebrovascular disease, documented by any one of the following: • CVA: Patient has a history of stroke (ie, loss of neurologic function with residual symptoms at least 24 h after onset) presumed to be from vascular cause • Transient ischemic attack (TIA): Patient has a history of loss of neurologic function that was abrupt in onset but with complete return of function within 24 h, presumed to be from vascular cause
13	Other comorbidities: diabetes	Patient has a history of diabetes diagnosed and/or treated by a physician; do not include gestational diabetes
14	FEV$_{1\%}$	FEV$_1$ obtained for the patient within 6 mo of the operation and expressed as percentage of the predicted for age, sex, and height according to the prediction equations (after bronchodilators if done)
15	DLCO%	Uncorrected DLCO obtained for the patient within 6 mo of the operation and expressed as percentage of the predicted for age, sex, and height according to prediction equations
16	ECOG: Zubrod	The Zubrod performance scale should be marked to indicate the level of the patient's performance at the time of operation that most accurately defines the patient's status
17	Diagnosis: lung cancer (NSCLC)	Indicate whether a lung resection was performed for lung cancer (eg, wedge, segment, lobe, pneumonectomy), open or VATS

(continued on next page)

Table 2
(continued)

	Variable	Definition
18	Clinic T	Appropriate descriptor for the primary tumor according to the 7th edition of the AJCC lung cancer staging system; clinical staging is based on the pretreatment estimated (before any induction therapy is done) staging workup, which may include, for instance, CT scan, PET scan, endoscopic ultrasonography
19	cN	Appropriate descriptor for the lung cancer nodal metastases according to the 7th edition of the AJCC lung cancer staging system; all nodes >1 cm on CT or PET/CT are considered positive; all PET-positive nodes are considered positive; results of previous invasive staging (EBUS, mediastinoscopy) should be included here; clinical staging is based on the pretreatment estimated (before any induction therapy is done) staging workup, which may include, for instance, CT scan, PET scan, endoscopic ultrasonography
20	cM	Appropriate descriptor for the lung cancer distant metastases according to the 7th edition of the AJCC lung cancer staging system; clinical staging is based on the pretreatment estimated (before any induction therapy is done) staging workup, which may include, for instance, CT scan, PET scan, endoscopic ultrasonography
21	Date of thoracic surgical procedure	Date of surgical procedure, which equals the date the patient enters the operating room
22	Status	Status that best describes the clinical status of the patient at the time of the primary surgical procedure: 1. Emergent: the surgical procedure must be performed without delay; the patient has no choice other than immediate operation if he or she does not want to risk permanent disability or death. 2. Urgent: the surgical procedure can wait until the patient is medically stable but should generally be done within 48 h. 3. Elective: surgical procedure that is scheduled in advance because it does not involve a medical emergency
23	ASA	Patient's ASA Risk Scale for this surgical procedure
24	pT	Appropriate descriptor for the lung cancer primary tumor based on final pathology report according to the 7th edition of the AJCC lung cancer staging system
25	pN	Appropriate descriptor for the lung cancer regional nodes based on final pathology report according to the 7th edition of the AJCC lung cancer staging system
26	pM	Appropriate descriptor for the lung cancer metastases based on final pathology report according to the 7th edition of the AJCC lung cancer staging system
27	pR	Pathology report indicated positive surgical margins
28	Complication: air leak >5 d	Patient experienced a postoperative air leak for >5 d
29	Complication: bronchoscopy for atelectasis	Postoperative atelectasis documented clinically or radiographically that needed bronchoscopy
30	Complication: pneumonia	Defined according to the last CDC criteria: 2 or more serial chest radiographs with at least *1* of the following: 1. New or progressive *and* persistent infiltrate 2. Consolidation 3. Cavitation *and* at least *1* of the following: 1. Fever (>38°C or >100.4°F) with no other recognized cause 2. Leukopenia (<4000 WBC/mm^3) or leukocytosis ($\geq$12,000 WBC/mm^3) 3. For adults $\geq$70 years old, altered mental status with no other recognized cause

(continued on next page)

Table 2
(continued)

	Variable	Definition
		and at least *2* of the following:
		1. New onset of purulent sputum, or change in character of sputum, or increased respiratory secretions, or increased suctioning requirements
		2. New onset or worsening cough, or dyspnea, or tachypnea
		3. Rales or bronchial breath sounds
		Worsening gas exchange (eg, O_2 desaturations (eg, Pao_2/Fio_2 $\leq$240), increased oxygen requirements, or increased ventilator demand)
31	Complication: ARDS	ARDS defined according to the American-European consensus conference; all of the following criteria should be met:
		1. Acute onset
		2. Arterial hypoxemia with Pao_2/Fio_2 ratio <200 (regardless of PEEP level)
		3. Bilateral infiltrates at chest radiograph or CT scan
		4. No clinical evidence of left atrial hypertension or pulmonary artery occlusive pressure <18 mm Hg
		5. Compatible risk factors
32	Complication: bronchopleural fistula	Patient experienced a complete or partial dehiscence of the bronchial stump documented in the postoperative period (such as bronchoscopy or other operative intervention)
33	Complication: pulmonary embolism	Patient experienced a pulmonary embolus in the postoperative period as documented by a V/Q scan, angiogram, or spiral CT
34	Complication: initial ventilator support >48 h	Patient initially was ventilated >48 h in the postoperative period; ventilator support ends with removal of endotracheal tube or, if the patient has a tracheostomy tube, until no longer ventilator dependent
35	Complication: reintubation	Patient was reintubated during the initial hospital stay after the initial extubation; this may include patients who have been extubated in the operating room and require intubation in the postoperative period
36	Complication: tracheostomy	Patient required a tracheostomy in the postoperative period whether performed in the ICU or the OR; prophylactic minitracheostomy on the day of operation should not be considered a complication
37	Complication: atrial arrhythmia	New onset of atrial fibrillation/flutter (AF) requiring medical treatment or cardioversion; does not include recurrence of AF that was present preoperatively
38	Complication: ventricular arrhythmia	Sustained ventricular tachycardia or ventricular fibrillation that has been clinically documented and treated by ablation therapy, implantable cardioverter defibrillator, permanent pacemaker, pharmacologic treatment. or cardioversion
39	Complication: myocardial infarction	Evidenced by 1 of the following criteria:
		1. Transmural infarction diagnosed by the appearance of a new Q wave in 2 or more contiguous leads on ECG
		2. Subendocardial infarction (non Q wave) evidenced by clinical, angiographic, electrocardiographic signs
		3. Laboratory isoenzyme evidence of myocardial necrosis
40	Complication: empyema	Patient experienced an empyema requiring treatment in the postoperative period; diagnosis of empyema should be confirmed by thoracentesis; frank pus or merely cloudy fluid may be aspirated from the pleural space; the pleural fluid typically has leukocytosis, low pH (<7.20), low glucose (<60 mg/dL), high lactate dehydrogenase, and elevated protein and may contain infectious organisms
41	Complication: wound infection	Patient experienced a wound infection in the postoperative period as evidenced by meeting 2 of the following criteria:
		1. Wound opened with excision of tissue (I&D)
		2. Positive culture
		3. Treatment with antibiotics

(continued on next page)

Table 2
(continued)

	Variable	Definition
42	Complication: cerebrovascular complications	Occurrence of 1 of the following central neurologic postoperative events not present preoperatively: 1. A central neurologic deficit persisting postoperatively for more than 72 h 2. A transient neurologic deficit (TIA or reversible ischemic neurologic deficit) with recovery within 72 h 3. A new postoperative coma persisting at least 24 h and caused by anoxic/ischemic and/or metabolic encephalopathy, thromboembolic event, or cerebral bleed
43	Complication: recurrent nerve palsy	Patient experienced in the postoperative period a recurrent laryngeal nerve paresis or paralysis that was not identified during the preoperative evaluation
44	Complication: delirium	Patient experienced a new onset of symptoms like illusions, confusion, cerebral excitement in the postoperative period
45	Complication: renal failure	Defined as the onset of new renal failure in the postoperative period according to 1 of the following criteria: 1. Increase of serum creatinine to >2.0 mg/dL 2. Two times the preoperative creatinine level 3. A new requirement for dialysis postoperatively
46	Complication: chylothorax	Patient experienced a chylothorax in the postoperative period that required persistent or new drainage and medical intervention (eg, NPO, TPN) or reoperation. Chylothorax is defined by the clinical appearance of the pleural fluid or the presence of pleural fluid triglyceride levels >110 mg/dL with a cholesterol level <200 mg/dL
47	Complication: unexpected admission to ICU	An unplanned transfer of the patient to the ICU owing to deterioration in the condition of the patient requiring active life support treatment
48	Date of discharge	Date the patient was discharged from the hospital (acute care); if the patient died in the hospital, the discharge date is the date of death
49	Outcome at discharge	Indicate whether patient was alive or dead at discharge from the hospitalization in which the primary surgical procedure occurred
50	Outcome at 30 d	Indicate whether patient was alive or dead 30 d after operation (whether in the hospital or not)

Abbreviations: AJCC, American Joint Committee on Cancer; ARDS, adult respiratory distress syndrome; ASA, American Society of Anesthesiologists; CABG, coronary artery bypass grafting; CDC, Centers for Disease Control and Prevention; CT, computed tomography; CV, cardiovascular; CVA, cerebrovascular accident; EBUS, endobronchial ultrasonography; ECG, electrocardiogram; ECOG, Eastern Cooperative Oncology Group; FEV_1, forced expiratory volume in 1 second; I&D, incision and drainage; ICU, intensive care unit; NPO, nothing by mouth; NSCLC, non–small-cell lung cancer; OR, operating room; PCI, percutaneous coronary intervention; PEEP, positive end-expiratory pressure; TPN, total parenteral nutrition; VATS, video-assisted thoracic surgery; WBC, white blood cells.

From Fernandez FG, Falcoz PE, Kozower BD, et al. The Society of Thoracic Surgeons and the European Society of Thoracic Surgeons General Thoracic Surgery Databases: joint standardization variable definitions terminology. Ann Thorac Surg 2015;99:368–76.

representatives from both societies proposed a definition and, after comparison and revision, they provided a standardized agreed-on definition. This effort was reported in a comprehensive review outlining the history and aims of the databases, the newly defined common terminology, and agreed-on definitions.[15] For example, a standardized definition of wound infection in the postoperative period was agreed on as meeting 2 of the following criteria: wound opened with excision of tissue, positive culture, or treatment with antibiotics.

Harmonization of the databases allowed the first project comparing data from the STS GTSD and ESTS registry.[15] Between 2010 and 2013, 78,212 (STS, 47,539; ESTS, 30,673) patients who underwent pulmonary resection were compared for variation in treatment

Table 3
Common definitions of variables not present in both databases

Variable	Definition
Peripheral vascular disease	Indicate whether the patient has peripheral arterial vascular disease, as indicated by • Claudication with either exertion or rest • Amputation for arterial insufficiency • Aortoiliac occlusive disease reconstruction • Peripheral vascular bypass procedure, angioplasty, or stent • Documented AAA, AAA repair, or stent • Noninvasive/invasive carotid test with >79% occlusion • Previous carotid artery surgical procedure or intervention for carotid artery stenosis
Pulmonary hypertension	• Right heart catheterization: mean pulmonary arterial pressure (PAP) >25 mm Hg at rest or • Echocardiographic diagnosis: tricuspid regurgitation velocity 3.4 m/s, pulmonary artery systolic pressure >50 mm Hg
COPD	GOLD American Thoracic Society definition • No: $FEV_1/FVC \geq 0.7$ • Mild: $FEV_1/FVC < 0.7$ and $FEV_1 \geq 80\%$ • Moderate: $FEV_1/FVC < 0.7$ and $80\% < FEV_1 > 50\%$ • Severe: $FEV_1/FVC < 0.7$ and $FEV_1 < 50\%$
Pulmonary fibrosis	Indicate whether the patient has a diagnosis of interstitial fibrosis based on clinical and radiologic or pathologic evidence
Readmission	Indicate whether patient was readmitted to any hospital within 30 d of discharge because of any cause related to previous operation
FVC (L)	FVC: the amount of air (expressed in liters) that can be forcibly exhaled from the lungs after taking the deepest breath possible
FVC%	Forced vital capacity: the amount of air (expressed as percentage of theoretic value) in liters that can be forcibly exhaled from the lungs after taking the deepest breath possible
FEV_1 (L)	Forced expiratory volume in 10 second: the amount of air (expressed in liters) that can be forcibly exhaled from the lungs in the first second of a forced exhalation
FEV_1/FVC (L)	The number that represents the ratio of forced expiratory volume in 1 s (FEV_1) to forced vital capacity (FVC)
ppoFEV$_1$%	Predicted postoperative FEV_1 is calculated taking into account the number of functioning segments to be resected during operation (ppoFEV$_1$ = preoperative $FEV_1 \times [1 - a/b]$), where a = number of unobstructed segments to be resected and b = total number of unobstructed segments, according to the ERS/ESTS and ACCP guidelines
ppoDLCO%	Predicted postoperative DLCO is calculated taking into account the number of functioning segments to be resected during operation (ppoDLCO = preoperative DLCO $\times [1 - a/b]$), where a = number of unobstructed segments to be resected and b = total number of unobstructed segments, according to the ERS/ESTS and ACCP guidelines
Vo_{2max}	Vo_{2max} is the maximal oxygen uptake or the maximum volume of oxygen that can be used in 1 min during maximal or exhaustive exercise; it is measured as milliliters of oxygen used in 1 min per kilogram of body weight

Although the ESTS-STS Task Force agreed on a common definition of variables that are currently not present in both datasets, their inclusion in future versions or upgrades of the 2 databases will depend on each individual database committee decision.

Abbreviations: AAA, abdominal aortic aneurysm; ACCP, American College of Chest Physicians; COPD, chronic obstructive pulmonary disease; DLCO, diffusing capacity of the lungs for carbon monoxide; ERS, European Respiratory Society; ESTS, European Society of Thoracic Surgeons; FEV_1, forced expiratory volume in 1 second; FVC, forced vital capacity; GOLD, generalized obstructive lung disease; STS, Society of Thoracic Surgeons.

From Fernandez FG, Falcoz PE, Kozower BD, et al. The Society of Thoracic Surgeons and the European Society of Thoracic Surgeons General Thoracic Surgery Databases: joint standardization variable definitions terminology. Ann Thorac Surg 2015;99:368–76.

practices and short-term outcomes. This analysis revealed that a larger proportion of patients in the STS GTSD were women, had undergone previous cardiothoracic surgery, and had preoperative thoracic radiation. In addition, patients in the STS GTSD had higher American Society of Anesthesiologists classifications and Zubrod scores, consistent with the greater incidence of comorbidities, including obesity, hypertension, congestive heart failure, and coronary artery disease. Thoracoscopic procedures (62.5% vs 21.8%; P<.001) and sublobar resections (43.3% vs 31.1%; P<.001) were significantly more common in the STS GTSD, despite a similar proportion of surgeries performed for primary lung cancer. In addition, fewer patients were found to have pathologic N2 or M1 disease at the time of surgery in the STS GTSD than the ESTS registry.

Examining outcomes between the databases, the STS GTSD demonstrated a shorter median hospital length of stay, despite reporting more frequent reintubation and atrial arrhythmias. Thirty-day mortality was higher in the STS GTSD for patients who underwent wedge resection (1.9% vs 0.1%; P<.05). Conversely, STS GTSD mortality was lower for lobectomy (1.4% vs 2.6%; P<.05) and pneumonectomy (4.9% vs 7.3%; P<.05) compared with the ESTS Database.

Although some intersocietal variation is expected due to regional influences and lack of risk adjustment, differences in outcomes suggest the opportunity for quality improvement initiatives. This study acts as a basis for future investigation, potentially examining stage-specific, risk-adjusted outcomes to better understand causes of intersocietal variation. The STS GTSD is actively working to collect long-term outcome data at the institutional level and is in the process of linking with governmental claims databases.[17] As more long-term follow-up data become available, comparisons of intersocietal variation will become increasingly informative.

CHALLENGES IN COLLABORATION

As the STS GTSD and the ESTS registry Task Forces have developed a common interest in designing studies based on the use of shared data derived from the registries, certain challenges have arisen. The process of merging databases, before data mining, is a fundamental and complex step. To facilitate the creation of common datasets, the STS GTSD and ESTS registry Task Forces have harmonized many variables, with the aim of obtaining shared and standardized definitions for the most common variables collected.[15] However, despite this harmonization, additional technical barriers must be overcome during the development of each study. The creation of an "ad hoc" dataset is conditional on specific steps during the data transformation phase:

- Identification of the items/variables of interest
- Validation of the variables homogeneity (definition, unit of measure, limits)
- Confirmation of the syntax for each variable
- Definition and check of the completeness level for each variable
- Creation of data transfer agreements between societies
- Creation of a new data repository
- Maintenance of the derived base of data
- Societal agreement on interpretation of results.

These activities have been carried out for the common studies performed by the 2 societies, preliminary to the analysis of data. Perhaps in the future, the STS GTSD and the ESTS Database Task Forces could work together to optimize methodology for creating a shared database available for agreed-on international projects. To ensure high data quality, such an intersocietal data repository should be validated by data quality assessment procedures using specific data quality indicators. Hopefully, standardized methods for measuring and improving the data quality in multi-institutional and international registries will be jointly developed by the 2 societies and applied in future studies.

FUTURE DIRECTIONS

The STS GTSD and ESTS registry Task Forces hold a joint session at the Society of Thoracic Surgeons Annual Conference each year, during which future projects are proposed and discussed. The possibilities are numerous, but ongoing efforts may include working toward complete synchronization between the STS GTSD and the ESTS registry. Although many variables were harmonized initially,[15] there still remain discrepancies. This would facilitate future studies that pool data from both societies or potentially allow intercontinental validation of risk models.

One project currently under way includes the pooling of STS GTSD and ESTS registry data to examine the hypothesis that surgical resection, including pneumonectomy, when performed as part of a multimodality regimen for stage IIIA (N2) non–small-cell lung cancer, is associated with low rates of perioperative morbidity and mortality. Pooling data from the STS GTSD and the ESTS registry provides the ideal opportunity to generate large-scale, meaningful, current perioperative outcome data that may differ from historical data and have a significant impact on clinical practice.

Other potential projects could include the transatlantic validation of societal risk models or even creation of "international" or "world" risk models for short-term morbidity and mortality. Alternatively, collaboration between the societal database Task Forces sets the stage for Delphi processes investigating best care practices in general thoracic surgery, potentially identifying quality endpoints to be used for international credentialing purposes. Currently, the STS is moving away from process measures as quality indicators, whereas the ESTS uses process measure to calculate performance scores for European institutional accreditation.

Finally, collaboration with other international databases remains an interest of the STS GTSD and ESTS registry Task Forces. These partnerships will make more data available for examination and provide international perspectives, with the universal goal of improving the quality of care for general thoracic surgical patients worldwide.

SUMMARY

In conclusion, international database collaboration between the STS GTSD and the ESTS registry Task Forces has been a fruitful and productive endeavor. Starting with the identification for the need to harmonize key variables in both databases, this partnership has ultimately led to multiple publications. Future projects are planned, with the overarching goal of improving quality of care for thoracic surgical patients worldwide. To that end, development of new partnerships with additional international databases will likely be pursued as time goes on.

REFERENCES

1. Wright CD, Edwards FH. The Society of Thoracic Surgeons General Thoracic Surgery Database. Ann Thorac Surg 2007;83(3):893–4.
2. Seder CW, Wright CD, Chang AC, et al. The Society of Thoracic Surgeons General Thoracic Surgery Database update on outcomes and quality. Ann Thorac Surg 2016;101(5):1646–54.
3. Magee MJ, Wright CD, McDonald D, et al. External validation of the Society of Thoracic Surgeons General Thoracic Surgery Database. Ann Thorac Surg 2013;96(5):1734–9.
4. The National Quality Forum. 2016. Available at: http://www.qualityforum.org/Home.aspx. Accessed September 19, 2016.
5. Fernandez FG, Kosinski A, Burfeind W, et al. STS lung cancer resection risk model: higher quality data and superior outcomes. Ann Thorac Surg 2016;102(2):370–7.
6. Raymond DP, Seder CW, Wright CD, et al. Predictors of major morbidity or mortality after resection for esophageal cancer: a Society of Thoracic Surgeons General Thoracic Surgery Database Risk Adjustment Model. Ann Thorac Surg 2016;102(1):207–14.
7. Kozower BD, O'Brien SM, Kosinski AS, et al. The Society of Thoracic Surgeons composite score for rating program performance for lobectomy for lung cancer. Ann Thorac Surg 2016;101(4):1379–86.
8. Society of Thoracic Surgeons General Thoracic Surgery Database Task Force. The Society of Thoracic Surgeons composite score for evaluating esophagectomy for esophageal cancer. Ann Thorac Surg 2017. [Epub ahead of print].
9. Berrisford R, Brunelli A, Rocco G, et al, on behalf of the Audit Guidelines Committee of the European Association for Cardiothoracic Surgery and the European Society of Thoracic Surgeons. The European Thoracic Surgery Database project: modeling the risk of in-hospital death following lung resection. Eur J Cardiothorac Surg 2005;28:306–11.
10. Brunelli A, Varela G, Van Schil P, et al. Multicentric analysis of performance after major lung resections by using the European Society Objective Score (ESOS). Eur J Cardiothorac Surg 2008;33:284–8.
11. Brunelli A, Berrisford RG, Rocco G, et al. European Society of Thoracic Surgeons Database Committee. The European Thoracic Database project: composite performance score to measure quality of care after major lung resection. Eur J Cardiothorac Surg 2009;35:769–74.
12. Brunelli A, Rocco G, Van Raemdonck D, et al. Lessons learned from the European thoracic surgery database: the composite performance score. Eur J Surg Oncol 2010;36:S93–9.
13. Salati M, Brunelli A, Dahan M, et al, on behalf of the European Society of Thoracic Surgeons Database Committee. Task-independent metrics to assess the data quality of medical registries using the European Society of Thoracic Surgeons (ESTS) Database. Eur J Cardiothorac Surg 2011;40:91–8.
14. Salati M, Falcoz PE, Decaluwe H, et al, on behalf of the ESTS Database Committee. The European thoracic data quality project: an aggregate data quality score to measure the quality of international multi-institutional databases. Eur J Cardiothorac Surg 2016;49:1470–5.
15. Fernandez FG, Falcoz PE, Kozower BD, et al. The Society of Thoracic Surgeons and The European

Society of Thoracic Surgeons General Thoracic Surgery Databases: joint standardization variable definitions terminology. Ann Thorac Surg 2015;99: 368–76.

16. Seder CW, Salati M, Kozower BD, et al. Variation in pulmonary resection practices between the Society of Thoracic Surgeons and European Society of Thoracic Surgeons General Thoracic Surgery Databases. Ann Thorac Surg 2016;101(6):2077–84.

17. Fernandez FG, Furnary AP, Kosinski AS, et al. Longitudinal follow-up of lung cancer resection from the Society of Thoracic Surgeons General Thoracic Surgery database in patients 65 years and older. Ann Thorac Surg 2016;101(6):2067–76.

Hospital Readmission Following Thoracic Surgery

Richard K. Freeman, MD, MBA

KEYWORDS

• Quality • Readmission • Lobectomy • Esophagectomy

KEY POINTS

- Hospital readmission costs the health care system in excess of 1 billion dollars a year.
- The Hospital Readmission Reduction Program was instituted as part of the Affordable Care Act in 2012 and penalizes hospitals with high rates of readmission.
- Strategies exist to minimize hospital readmissions and should be implemented by thoracic surgeons.

In 2010, there were more than 35 million hospital discharges in the United States.[1] Among Medicare patients, nearly 20% who are discharged from a hospital are readmitted within 30 days.[2] Unplanned readmissions account for 17% of hospital payments from Medicare in 2004, which equates to 1.4 billion dollars a year. Although many readmissions are unavoidable, researchers have found wide variation in hospitals' readmission rates, suggesting that patients admitted to certain hospitals are more likely to experience readmissions compared with other hospitals.[3]

In an attempt to reduce preventable readmissions, the Centers for Medicare and Medicaid Services (CMS) initiated the Hospital Readmissions Reduction Program (HRRP) in 2012 authorized by the Affordable Care Act (ACA). This program reduced hospital reimbursement by up to 1% if the facility was found to have an above-average risk-adjusted readmission rates for conditions representing a high percentage of readmissions such as myocardial infarction, congestive heart failure, or pneumonia.

For 2017, 78% of Medicare patient admissions are projected to be in hospitals receiving either no readmission penalty or penalties of less than 1% of the hospital's Medicare inpatient payments. Fewer than 2% of Medicare patient admissions will be in hospitals receiving the maximum financial penalty. Total Medicare penalties assessed on hospitals for readmissions will increase to $528 million in 2017. This amount is $108 million more than seen in 2016 and is predominantly owing to more medical conditions being measured.

This review recounts the first 5 years of readmission efforts under the HRRP. Consideration is also given to the challenges of using readmissions as a surrogate metric for quality. An overview of readmission reduction strategies and resources is then outlined. Finally, a discussion of the future of the HRRP is provided.

THE HOSPITAL READMISSIONS REDUCTION PROGRAM

A hospital readmission occurs when a patient is admitted to a hospital within a specified period after being discharged from an earlier (initial) hospitalization. For Medicare, this period is defined as 30 days and includes hospital readmissions to

The author has no conflicts of interest to declare.
Department of Thoracic and Cardiovascular Surgery, St Vincent Hospital, 8433 Harcourt Road, Indianapolis, IN 46260, USA
E-mail address: Richard.Freeman@StVincent.org

any hospital, not just the hospital at which the patient was originally hospitalized. Medicare uses an all-cause definition of readmission. This definition means that hospital stays within 30 days of a discharge from an initial hospitalization are considered readmissions regardless of the reason for the readmission. This all-cause definition is used in calculating both the national average readmission rate and each hospital's specific readmission rate. Starting in 2014, CMS began making an exception for planned hospitalizations (such as a scheduled coronary angioplasty) within the 30-day window.

The HRRP was established by a provision in the ACA requiring Medicare to reduce payments to hospitals with relatively high readmission rates for patients in non–managed care Medicare. Starting in 2013, as a permanent component of Medicare's inpatient hospital payment system, the HRRP was applied to most acute care hospitals. Hospitals excluded were psychiatric, rehabilitation, long-term care, children's, cancer, and critical access hospitals. Under the HRRP, hospitals with readmission rates that exceed the national average are penalized by a reduction in payments across all of their Medicare admissions.

Before comparing a hospital's readmission rate with the national average, CMS adjusts for demographic characteristics of both the patients being readmitted and each hospital's patient population such as age and illness severity. After these adjustments, CMS calculates a rate of excess readmissions, which links directly to the hospital's readmission penalty in a progressive fashion.[4] Each year, CMS releases each hospital's penalty for the upcoming year in the Federal Register and posts this information on its Medicare Web site.

For fiscal year 2013, the maximum penalty was 1% of the hospital's base Medicare inpatient payments. This increased to 2% for 2014 and then 3% starting in 2015.[5] When calculating each hospital's readmission rate, CMS uses 3 full years of hospital data. Accordingly, the upcoming 2017 penalties are based on hospital readmissions that occurred from July 2012 through June 2015.

For penalties levied in 2013 and 2014, CMS focused on readmissions after initial hospitalizations for 3 selected conditions; heart attack, heart failure, and pneumonia.[6] Included conditions in 2015 added chronic obstructive pulmonary disease and elective hip or knee replacement. For 2017 penalties, CMS expanded the types of pneumonia cases that were assessed and added readmission rates following coronary artery bypass graft surgery.

CMS has been posting individual hospital readmission rates on its Hospital Compare Web site, in addition to other measures of quality and patient satisfaction, since 2009. Designed for use by Medicare consumers and researchers, this Web site also provides comparisons of each hospital's Medicare readmission performance to the national average by indicating whether the hospital is "better/worse/no different" than the US National rate. In addition to readmissions following hospitalizations for selected diagnoses, the Hospital Compare Web site reports each hospital's overall Medicare readmission rates.

Analysis of this database shows that 2012 marks the first measurable declines in readmissions. Specifically, when the 3-year running average of hospital readmission rates began including data from 2012, the rates decreased across all 3 diagnosis categories. This trend has continued through subsequent measurement periods.[7]

Regardless of whether a correct deduction, the reduction in hospital readmissions following the enactment of HRRP suggests that hospitals may have initiated new interventions to lower their readmission rates during the measurement period leading up to the fines. The Department of Health and Human Services estimates 565,000 fewer Medicare patient readmissions from April 2010 through May 2015.[8,9]

CURRENT STATE OF READMISSION PENALTIES FOR HOSPITALS

Analysis of the variation in penalties by type of hospital suggests that Medicare beneficiaries who go to certain types of hospitals, especially major teaching hospitals and hospitals with relatively greater shares of low-income patients, are more likely to continue to be penalized and at a higher rate than the average.[10]

To some degree, there is overlap among these 2 types of hospitals, as major teaching hospitals often serve as safety net hospitals with higher proportions of low-income patients. Across all years, hospitals with the smallest share of low-income beneficiaries are the least likely to be assessed any penalty at all. It is predicted that for 2017, 66% of hospitals in the lowest quartile of low-income patients will be fined a readmission penalty compared with 86% among hospitals with the highest share of low-income beneficiaries. Rural hospitals also have higher rates of being penalized and higher average penalties. Variations in penalty rates by hospital characteristics have persisted across all 5 years of the program.[7]

Although the CMS readmission measures are adjusted for demographic characteristics associated with higher rates of hospital readmissions (such as age), the initial HRRP statute did not allow adjustments to the penalty calculations based on socioeconomic or community-level factors. However, after recommendations by the National Quality Forum and the Medicare Payment Advisory Commission to adjust for socioeconomic status, Congress recently modified the method that CMS will use to assess hospital performance.[6]

Specifically, the new law directs the Secretary of Health and Human Services to divide hospitals into peer groups based on similar shares of inpatients who qualify for both Medicare and full Medicaid and then determine each hospital's performance on readmissions relative to its peer group. This change will be effective fiscal year 2019, but the law also allows for the Secretary to consider implementing additional risk adjustments in the future.

The Centers for Medicare and Medicaid has previously raised concerns regarding socioeconomic adjustment. Specifically, the potential that risk adjusting penalties for hospitals with lower-income patients could hold those hospitals to a lower standard and unintentionally weaken incentives to improve health outcomes for disadvantaged patients.[8] In part, the peer group methodology may address some of this concern. However, depending on how the hospital peer groups are segregated, further complicating issues could arise because of state variation in the criteria for Medicaid eligibility among seniors and people with disabilities.

Hospital performance in the HRRP is essentially graded on a curve because the calculations for determining penalties are based on comparisons to the national average. Therefore, for each measure, if the national rate of Medicare readmissions declines, it is possible for hospitals to improve their readmission rates but still be penalized. Furthermore, the shifting penalties do not capture hospital performance across all initial hospitalization diagnoses—referred to as a hospitalwide or all-condition readmission measure.

Some suggest that if Medicare established fixed target rates for an all-condition readmission measure, hospitals might have an easier time understanding the HRRP, embracing interventions to achieve those targets, and would not risk some readmissions being double counted (eg, in the case of coronary artery bypass grafting and heart failure).[6] On the other hand, others argue that a fixed target for all conditions might mitigate the level of hospital improvement because it would establish a minimum performance rather than encourage hospitals to keep up with the average for each of the selected diagnoses.

Hospital administrators and policymakers have noted that incentives to reduce readmissions should not rest on hospitals alone because other providers and the patients themselves may play important roles in this effort. Further, hospitals may have little to no control over the care that patients receive after they are discharged from an inpatient stay. Although researchers readily acknowledge that many readmissions are not preventable, studies show that hospitals can engage in collaborative activities to lower their numbers of readmissions, such as clarifying patient discharge instructions, coordinating with post–acute care providers, and reducing medical complications during the patients' initial hospital stays.[11–14]

Not unexpectedly, there has been some disagreement with the hypothesis that readmission rates are a reflection of the quality of medical care provided to patients during an inpatient admission. Tsai and colleagues[15] using Medicare data for surgical procedures including coronary artery bypass and pulmonary lobectomy found "surgical readmission rates have a modest but consistent relationship with measures of surgical quality."

However, several studies have identified patient-level factors, such as patient age and severity of underlying illness or length of stay that are independently predictive of readmission.[16–20] Gale and colleagues[21] in a recent report in Health Affairs found that 30-day readmission rates don't reflect clear quality differences from one hospital to another. The authors found that readmissions occurring 7 days or more beyond an initial discharge were explained by community and household-level factors. They suggested using shorter intervals of 5 or 7 days to improve the accuracy of readmissions as a quality measurement.

READMISSION FOR THORACIC SURGERY PATIENTS

With the preceding background in mind, one wonders what is in store for thoracic surgery patients regarding readmissions. Although thoracic surgery does not currently have a procedure identified as a readmission metric in the HRRP, one will likely be designated in the coming years of the program. When the frequency and cost of thoracic surgical procedures are reviewed, the most likely metrics would seem to be lobectomy of the lung.

However, until recently, readmission to the hospital following most thoracic surgical procedures was not routinely reported in the literature. The Society of Thoracic Surgeons' General Thoracic Surgical database does track readmissions. However, readmissions may be underestimated if patients are admitted to facilities other than the hospital sponsoring the database.[22]

Some recent literature does exist outlining the frequency, causes, and opportunities for pulmonary resection and readmission. Handy and colleagues[23] published one of the first modern reports of readmission following pulmonary resection in 2001. This investigation found that the overall readmission rate was 18.9% with a significant percentage of patients requiring more than one readmission.

Our own investigation found that readmission rates, as well as other quality parameters, differed among the specialties of physicians performing lobectomy for lung cancer.[24] Specifically, lobectomy for lung cancer had a higher rate of readmission and longer mean length of stay when performed by a general surgeon compared with a cardiothoracic surgeon. Such information in the era of the HRRP program may have significant implications for the credentialing process at hospitals.

In a separate investigation, our group reported that mean length of stay after lobectomy is negatively associated with readmission rates, with the maximal effect being before postoperative day 5.[25] Furthermore, facility reimbursement was optimized when length of stay was extended to minimize the risk of readmission. This investigation did not take into account that the HRRP program began after this investigation.

In a well-designed study looking at readmission rates following lung resection for lung cancer, Hu and colleagues[22] reviewed the linked Surveillance, Epidemiology, and End Results (SEER)- Medicare database. The authors found a readmission rate of 12.8% with 28.3% of patients being readmitted to a facility other than the one at which surgery was performed. Factors associated with early readmission following lung cancer resection included patient comorbidities, type of operation, and socioeconomic factors. They also found that readmitted patients had an increased risk of death and demand maximum attention and optimal care.

There is less modern literature pertaining to readmission following the other complex procedure most often associated with thoracic surgery—esophagectomy. Sundaram and colleagues[26] found a readmission rate of 12.6% following esophagectomy in the NSQIP (National Surgery Quality Improvement Program) database. The most common reason for readmission was pulmonary complications with patients with pre-existing lung disease having an increased risk. These findings were confirmed by Chen and colleagues[27] in a similarly designed study.

Hu and colleagues[28] also collaborated on a linked SEER-Medicare database review of patients undergoing esophagectomy. In this investigation, they found a readmission rate of 20.7%. Readmission following esophagectomy was associated with a

4-fold increase in mortality rate. Multivariable regression found that readmission was the strongest predictor of mortality (odds ratio, 6.64; $P<.001$), with a stronger association than age, Charlson score, and index length of stay. Readmission diagnoses with the highest mortality rates were those associated with pulmonary, gastrointestinal, and cardiovascular diagnoses.

Realizing that even with the previously outlined potential inaccuracies inherent in measuring readmissions, the HRRP is not likely to be discarded. It is also likely that the measured conditions/procedures will increase over time. Therefore, it is necessary for all practitioners, including thoracic surgeons, to invest in understanding the research and processes behind readmission prevention.

Several factors that increase the likelihood of readmission may be modifiable, especially those that relate to clinician or system-level issues. Such factors include premature discharge, inadequate postdischarge support, insufficient follow-up, therapeutic errors, adverse drug events and other medication related issues, failed handoffs, complications following procedures, nosocomial infections, pressure ulcers, and patient falls.

Medical errors are a major contributor to preventable readmissions. Medication-related errors are estimated to occur in approximately 20% of patients following discharge.[29,30] Approximately two-thirds of such adverse events were determined to be either preventable or ameliorable. Examples of medication errors include patients sent home without prescriptions for necessary medications, patients receiving duplicate prescriptions for medications they have at home labeled with a different name (generic and proprietary names), inadequate monitoring, and follow-up for drug side effects.

However, preventing medication errors after discharge is challenging. In a randomized trial involving 2 tertiary care hospitals, an intervention involving pharmacist medication reconciliation at hospital discharge, pharmacist counseling, low-literacy aids, and postdischarge follow-up phone calls did not prevent clinically important medication errors. These errors occurred in one-half of patients in both the control and intervention groups.[31] Unfortunately, almost a quarter of these errors were serious with 13% leading to readmission or emergency department visits.

Poor information transfer, the so called failed handoff from hospital-based providers to primary care providers, occurs commonly. This finding may contribute to multiple adverse consequences, including the need for readmission, temporary or permanent disability, or death.[29,30,32] Tests that are pending at discharge often fail to be communicated to providers responsible for their follow-up.[33–35]

Findings reported in the literature include a study by Roy and colleagues,[33] which found that 41% of discharged patients had a test pending at discharge. Almost 1 in 10 of these patients potentially required an intervention. However, almost two-thirds of responsible aftercare providers were unaware that a test was outstanding. Similarly, Kripalani and colleagues[35] found tests pending at the time of discharge were mentioned in discharge summaries only 25% of the time, and the list of pending studies was complete only 13% of the time. Tests ordered on the day of discharge represent 7% of tests performed during hospitalization but account for 47% of tests that are never reviewed.[36] Another almost one-third of tests recommended by the hospital-based team for follow-up were never obtained by the aftercare provider.[37]

Unfortunately, direct communication from hospital provider to aftercare provider is uncommon. A meta-analysis found that only 12% to 34% of discharge summaries had reached aftercare providers by the time of the first posthospitalization appointment.[32] Additionally, the discharge documentation was often inaccurate and lacked important information such as noting additional workup indicated following discharge.

Follow-up care can also be confusing and executed in a less than optimal manner. The optimal interval between hospital discharge and the first follow-up visit to a primary care or subspecialty provider varies with the disease process and the patient. Many factors will contribute to this decision including the severity of the disease process being followed, the perceived ability of the patient to provide adequate self-care, and psychosocial and logistical factors. Among Medicare beneficiaries requiring readmission within 30 days of discharge, only 50% had seen a clinician for a follow-up visit.[2]

Several studies have evaluated the association between rates of readmission and scheduled outpatient follow-up posthospitalization. However, these studies are often complicated by 2 issues—many patients are readmitted before their scheduled follow-up visit and many of these studies exclude patients without established outpatient providers. Additionally, none of these studies are randomized trials.

Several studies affirm that patients who are scheduled or seen for posthospital follow-up are less likely to be readmitted.[30,38–40] A study of Medicare patients hospitalized for heart failure in 225 hospitals found that rates of readmission within 30 days were highest for patients discharged from the quartile of hospitals with the lowest percentage of patients seen for follow-up within 7 days of discharge.[38] Another observational study in a single academic primary care practice found that compared with patients in a faculty primary care practice, patients in resident primary care practices had lower rates of timely postdischarge follow-up and higher rates of readmission.[41] However, the study also noted differences in patients followed up by faculty practices and resident practices; patients followed up by residents were less likely to follow up with their primary provider and were more likely to be younger, African American, and covered by Medicaid.

By contrast, other studies have not found that scheduled outpatient follow-up decreases readmissions. One retrospective study of nearly 5000 hospital discharges from the general medicine service at the Mayo Clinic hospitals found no difference in 30-day hospital admission, emergency department visits, or mortality comparing patients who had documentation of a scheduled follow-up appointment (median 6 days after discharge) with those who did not.[42] This study, however, did not document whether those patients had actually attended the follow-up appointments or whether attending the follow-up visit resulted in changes in outcomes. In another study of 3661 patients age $\geq$65 years, there was no protective effect on readmission for patients who had a follow-up office visit within 7 days after discharge.[43]

Efforts to prevent readmissions can be targeted to patients known to be at a higher risk for readmission, including those at higher risk for adverse events postdischarge. But how are these patients identified? Studies suggest clinical and demographic parameters that may increase the risk of readmission. However, risk factors may not be the same for all readmissions. A cohort study at a single institution found that risk factors for early readmissions (within 1 week after discharge) were somewhat different than risk factors for later readmissions (between 8 and 30 days after discharge).[44–48]

Clinical factors include the following: the use of high-risk medication (antibiotics, glucocorticoids, anticoagulants, narcotics, antiepileptic medications, antipsychotics, antidepressants, and hypoglycemic agents),[38–40,49] polypharmacy (5 or more medications),[50] more than 6 chronic conditions[51] and certain specific clinical conditions (advanced chronic obstructive pulmonary disease, diabetes, heart failure, stroke, cancer, weight loss, depression).[52–58]

Demographic and logistical factors can also place a patient at increased risk for readmission.

Such conditions include unplanned hospitalizations within the last 6 to 12 months,[59–62] black race,[63,64] and a low level of health literacy.[65]

Reduced social network indicators like being alone most of the day with limited or no family or friend contact by phone or in person[62] was also found to be a factor as was a lower socioeconomic status.[66–68]

Studies have found that clinical providers are not able to accurately predict which patients will require readmission.[40] Screening for increased risk may help health care providers and organizations target resources to patients most likely to be rehospitalized. Several tools have now been developed and validated as methods for predicting readmission risk.

However, there are several caveats to the use of screening tools. Given the variability of resources, patient demographics, and case mix, it will be necessary to adjust risk prediction models for local factors. There will also be patients with very advanced disease or complicated social situations for whom no intervention will prevent readmission. Often efforts to decrease hospitalization are most effectively directed toward those patients with intermediate levels of risk for whom interventions might be successful.[69]

A guiding principle for using risk assessment is understanding how to implement interventions that target the risks identified. No screening tool will be perfectly accurate. Efforts to develop prediction models for patients at high risk for readmission have yielded only fair discriminative ability.[70,71] In a 2006 systematic review of 26 models developed to predict readmission, only one model focused on the prediction of preventable readmissions,[72] a concept that is fraught with issues regarding the definition of *preventability*.[73]

Screening tools that have been developed to identify patients at risk of readmission are of 2 types: risk scores and risk identifiers. Examples include the LACE index, which is a commonly used tool to identify patients at risk of readmission (not specifically potentially preventable readmission).[74] This model incorporates the patient's Length of stay, the Acuity of the patients admission, the degree of Comorbid illness (as measured by the Charlson Comorbidity Index), and the number of times the patients has been to the Emergency department in the last 6 months. The advantage of this model is the limited number of factors it includes. However, a limiting feature of LACE is that the length-of-stay element cannot be calculated accurately until the last day of the hospitalization.

The HOSPITAL score is another model specifically developed to identify avoidable readmissions.

Using a computerized, validated algorithm, the HOSPITAL score (calculated by points assigned for Hemoglobin less than 12 g/dL, discharge from the Oncology service, or Sodium less than 135 mEq/L at discharge; having a Procedure during the hospital stay; and Index admission Type: nonelective, number of hospital Admissions in the previous year, and Length of stay ≥5 days) identifies patients at high risk of 30-day potentially avoidable readmissions.[75] It was externally validated in a cohort study including more than 117,000 patients discharged from 9 hospitals across 4 different countries with moderately high discrimination.

Another tool for identifying patients at higher risk for readmission is the 8Ps Risk Assessment Tool, proposed by the Society of Hospital Medicine.[52] The 8Ps Risk Assessment Tool identifies risk factors for adverse events following hospital discharge. The 8 risk factors are similar to those clinical, demographic, and logistical factors described above. The 8Ps are a risk identification system rather than a risk score. However, the intent is that each risk identified will be matched with a risk-specific intervention.

Not surprisingly, patients who are discharged against medical advice are also higher-risk patients. A large retrospective cohort analysis performed at an urban academic medical center found that patients who were discharged against medical advice had a higher rate of readmission (odds ratio, 1.8; 95% confidence interval, 1.69–2.01) and also a 2-fold increased risk of death, compared with those discharged by their physician.[76] An against-medical-advice discharge was also more likely to occur for admissions related to substance abuse, sickle cell disease, or human immunodeficiency virus infection.

INTERVENTIONS TO REDUCE READMISSIONS

Efforts to re-engineer the discharge process to assure a safe transition involve issues such as improved clinician communication, patient education, information technology systems, involvement of community-based providers, and arrangements for prompt follow-up. Such interventions have the potential to substantially improve patient care and reduce health care expenditures as previously discussed.

A 2011 systematic review of 43 studies by Hansen and colleagues,[77] 16 of which were randomized trials, found that only 5 of the 16 randomized trials showed significant decreases in readmission rates. Four of the 5 successful studies involved several simultaneous interventions, including patient-centered discharge instructions and a post-discharge telephone call.

Similarly, a 2012 systematic review found that many types of interventions (including medication reconciliation, structured electronic discharge summaries, discharge planning, and facilitated communication between hospital and community providers) impacted favorably on outcomes including readmission rates.[78] However, because of heterogeneity in interventions, patient populations, and outcomes, it was not possible to identify which specific interventions had direct impact on measured outcomes.

A 2014 meta-analysis of 42 randomized trials found that tested interventions prevented early readmissions.[79] Mistiaen and Poot[80] found that the more effective interventions were those that were complex, multifaceted, and supported patients' capacity for self-care. Such multidisciplinary initiatives, often known as disease management programs, have targeted patients with specific chronic diseases to provide patient support, counseling, monitoring, and medication oversight through the continuum of care, including ambulatory, hospital, and hospital discharge settings.

Multiple investigations looked at the impact of a telephone call from a member of the health care team following discharge on varying parameters of patient management. These calls have been initiated by various members of the care team, including the discharging clinician, a clinical pharmacist, and a clinician from the patient's primary care clinic, nurses, nurse practitioners, and physician assistants.

Such calls have been moderately effective at reducing emergency department visits and improving follow-up with ambulatory providers but showed a trend toward reduced hospital readmissions in only 1 study.[81–83]

A 2006 systematic review was unable to define a clear benefit from postdischarge telephone calls because of significant heterogeneity in the quality and design of the investigations in this literature.[80] Interestingly, the optimal origin of the postdischarge telephone follow-up (hospital based or ambulatory based) is also unknown. A systematic review of the literature examining the effect of a telephone follow-up initiated by the primary care provider found no change in readmission rates, but the intervention did improve rates of postdischarge follow-up with the primary care practice.[84]

Home visits made by several different types of providers have also been shown to reduce the need for readmission. A report by Jerant and colleagues[85] illustrated that a single home visit by a

nurse and pharmacist to patients discharged with a diagnosis of heart failure with a goal of optimizing medication management, showed a trend toward an almost 50% reduced risk of unplanned readmission. Other studies looking at this question did not find as dramatic an effect on reduction in readmission.[86,87]

The use of telemonitoring devices has also been studied as a means for reducing readmissions. As an example, using an integrated telephonic stethoscope in conjunction with follow-up nursing calls in patients with heart failure reduced emergency department visits in one small study and showed a trend toward reduced readmissions and overall costs.[88] Devices for remotely monitoring various physiologic variables, including blood pressure, heart rate, weight, and oxygen saturation, have been repeatedly studied, mostly among heart failure patients, and have shown variable effectiveness in reducing need for readmission.[89]

As previously discussed, readmission may occur as a result of medication errors. Medication management may prevent readmissions. One single-center randomized trial in 278 patients on high-risk medications or greater than 3 medications on discharge compared usual care with medication management by a pharmacist (face-to-face medication reconciliation, patient-specific medication care plan, discharge counseling, and postdischarge telephone calls).[83] Patients who received medication management by a pharmacist were less likely to be readmitted or seen in the emergency department within 30 days of discharge. The results of this trial suggest that emergency department visit reduction was the larger driver of the primary outcome's composite elements. However, it does show the impact of clinical pharmacists and the importance of medication reconciliation in care transitions of hospitalized patients at discharge.

Given the complexity of transitions of care associated with hospital discharge, several studies have evaluated the effectiveness of multifaceted interventions in specific populations and health delivery environments. One such study evaluated the Care Transitions Intervention program in which older patients were paired with a discharge nurse transition coach. The transition coach facilitated self-management by the patient or a family caregiver instead of providing direct care.[13] The coach encouraged the patient to maintain a personal health record, obtain timely follow-up appointments, provide self-care, and understand what to do if problems arise. The transition coach saw the patient before discharge and at home 2 to 3 days after discharge, followed by 3 telephone calls over the first 28 days after discharge. This intervention reduced 30- and 90-day readmission rates significantly (8.3% vs 11.9% and 16.7% vs 22.5%, respectively) with a cost savings of approximately $500 per case.

Components of the Care Transitions Intervention program were implemented in the real-world setting of a sample of fee-for-service, English-speaking Medicare patients being discharged home for specific cardiac or respiratory conditions from 6 hospitals in Rhode Island.[90] Readmission rates within 30 days were lower for patients who received coaching compared with data from Medicare claims of an external control group of discharged patients with similar diagnoses who were not offered the intervention (odds ratio, 0.61; 95% confidence interval, 0.42–0.88).

A randomized trial in 6 geriatric inpatient units in France evaluated the effect of a multimodal intervention (comprehensive medication review; self-management education focusing on medications, depression, and nutrition; and detailed communication around transition of care) on readmission and emergency department visits.[91] Rates for these outcomes were lower at 3 months (a secondary outcome), but not at 6 months (the primary outcome), for the group assigned to the intervention. The intervention included implementation by a geriatrician dedicated to the project and thus might not be readily reproducible outside of the research project.

Another example of a targeted program to reduce readmissions is found in a randomized trial of 239 older adult patients with heart failure which compared assigned advanced practice nurses to coordinate discharge with standard, usual care.[92,93] The designated transitional care partner met with the patient daily during the index visit and made a home visit the day after discharge and at least weekly thereafter over the first 3 months. At 1 year, there were 104 readmissions among intervention patients compared with 162 readmissions for control patients, resulting in a cost savings of $4845 per patient.

Similarly, a prospective study of a nurse-led transitional care program for heart failure patients being discharged from one US hospital compared 30-day readmissions, length of stay, and 60-day direct costs with heart failure patients concurrently discharged from other hospitals within the same health care system.[94] The program was associated with a 48% decrease in 30-day readmissions. However, it had little impact on direct costs to the health care system over 60 days and had a negative impact on hospital revenue under the existing Medicare reimbursement system.

With the enactment of the HRRP in the ACA, the aim to reduce preventable hospital readmissions has gained traction among providers and policymakers. Moreover, key programs, such as Accountable Care Organizations, bundled payment initiatives, and medical home programs include provider incentives to lower hospital readmissions, either directly or indirectly. Additionally, the Community-based Care Transitions Program, also enacted by the ACA, is designed to assess ways that local organizations might partner with hospitals to improve patients' transitions to other settings, such as skilled nursing facilities or the patients' homes.[32,92–94] Also, in traditional Medicare, CMS has recently started allowing physicians to bill Medicare for transitional care management after a beneficiary's discharge from a hospital or other health care facility, in an effort to reimburse physicians for follow-up activities that could reduce readmissions and other complications.

FUTURE DIRECTIONS

All of these events make it unlikely that the focus on preventable hospital readmissions will diminish. For thoracic surgeons, several actions seem reasonable. The first is to be cognizant of readmissions in our own programs and to take actions to reduce them. Besides the list of tactics outlined, a list of other resources follow this discussion (Appendix 1).

On a more global note, we should encourage scholarly work related to thoracic surgical procedures to report readmission rates. As a specialty, thoracic surgery must increase participation in the Society of Thoracic Surgeons' General Thoracic Surgery Database. Such participation will eventually allow a critical mass of data to be accumulated, which will produce risk-adjusted data that are unrivaled in accuracy.

REFERENCES

1. Available at: http://www.cdc.gov/nchs/fastats/hospital.htm. Accessed January 26, 2016.
2. Jencks SF, Williams MV, Coleman EA. Rehospitalizations among patients in the Medicare fee-for-service program. N Engl J Med 2009;360(14):1418–28.
3. Epstein AM, Jha AK, Orav EJ, et al. The relationship between hospital admission rates and rehospitalizations. N Engl J Med 2011;365(24):2287–95.
4. Kahn C, Ault T, Potetz L, et al. Assessing Medicare's hospital pay-for-performance programs and whether they are achieving their goals. Health Aff (Millwood) 2015;34(8).
5. Joynt K, Jha A. A path forward on medicare readmissions. N Engl J Med 2013;368(13).
6. Medicare Payment Advisory Commission. Chapter 4: Refining the hospital readmissions reduction

program. Report to the Congress: Medicare and the Health Care Delivery System. 2013.

7. Zuckerman RS, Sheingold J, Orav J, et al. Readmissions, observations, and the hospital readmissions reduction program. N Engl J Med 2016;374(16): 1543–51.

8. Obama B. United States health care reform: progress to date and next steps. JAMA 2016;316(5): 525–32.

9. Final rule for 42 CFR parts 405, 412, 413. Fed Regist 2014;79(163):49659–50536.

10. Sheingold S, Zuckerman R, Shartzer A. Understanding Medicare hospital readmission rates and differing penalties between safety-net and other hospitals. Health Aff (Millwood) 2016;35(1).

11. Ahmad FS, Metlay JP, Barg FK, et al. Identifying hospital organizational strategies to reduce readmissions. Am J Med Qual 2013;28(4):278–85.

12. Silow-Carroll S, Edwards JN, Lashbrook A. "Reducing hospital readmissions: lessons from top-performing hospitals," Commonwealth Fund Synthesis Report. New York: Commonwealth Fund; 2011.

13. Jack BW, Chetty VK, Anthony D, et al. A reengineered hospital discharge program to decrease rehospitalization: a randomized trial. Ann Intern Med 2009;150(3):178–87.

14. Kanaan SB. Homeward bound: nine patient-centered programs cut readmissions. Oakland (CA): California HealthCare Foundation; 2009.

15. Tsai TC, Joynt KE, Orav EJ, et al. Variation in surgical-readmission rates and quality of hospital care. N Engl J Med 2013;369:1134–42.

16. Kassin MT, Owen RM, Perez SD, et al. Risk factors for 30-day hospital readmission among general surgery patients. J Am Coll Surg 2012;215:322–30.

17. Schneider EB, Hyder O, Brooke BS, et al. Patient readmission and mortality after colorectal surgery for colon cancer: impact of length of stay relative to other clinical factors. J Am Coll Surg 2012;214: 390–9.

18. Greenblatt DY, Greenberg CC, Kind AJ, et al. Causes and implications of readmission after abdominal aortic aneurysm repair. Ann Surg 2012; 256:595–605.

19. Vorhies JS, Wang Y, Herndon J, et al. Readmission and length of stay after total hip arthroplasty in a national Medicare sample. J Arthroplasty 2011;26(6 Suppl):119–23.

20. Hendren S, Morris AM, Zhang W, et al. Early discharge and hospital readmission after colectomy for cancer. Dis Colon Rectum 2011;54:1362–7.

21. Chin DL, Bang H, Manickam RN, et al. Rethinking thirty-day hospital readmissions: shorter intervals might be better indicators of quality of care. Health Aff (Millwood) 2016;35(10):1867–75.

22. Hu Y, McMurry TL, Isbell JM, et al. Readmission after lung cancer resection is associated with a 6-fold increase in 90-day postoperative mortality. J Thorac Cardiovasc Surg 2014;148:2261–7.

23. Handy JR Jr, Child AI, Grunkemeier GL, et al. Hospital readmission after pulmonary resection: prevalence, patterns, and predisposing characteristics. Ann Thorac Surg 2001;72:1855–9.

24. Freeman RK, Dilts JR, Ascioti AJ, et al. A comparison of quality and cost indicators by surgical specialty for lobectomy of the lung. J Thorac Cardiovasc Surg 2015;150(5):1254–60.

25. Freeman RK, Dilts JR, Ascioti AJ, et al. A comparison of length of stay, readmission rate, and facility reimbursement after lobectomy of the lung. Ann Thorac Surg 2013;96:1740–6.

26. Sundaram A, Srinivasan A, Baker S, et al. Readmission and risk factors for readmission following esophagectomy for esophageal cancer. J Gastrointest Surg 2015;19:581.

27. Chen SY, Molena D, Stem M, et al. Post-discharge complications after esophagectomy account for high readmission rates. World J Gastroenterol 2016;22(22):5246–53.

28. Hu Y, McMurry TL, Stukenborg GJ, et al. Readmission predicts 90-day mortality following esophagectomy: analysis of surveillance, epidemiology, and end results registry linked to -Medicare outcomes. J Thorac Cardiovasc Surg 2015;150(5):1254–60.

29. Forster AJ, Murff HJ, Peterson JF, et al. The incidence and severity of adverse events affecting patients after discharge from the hospital. Ann Intern Med 2003;138:161.

30. Forster AJ, Clark HD, Menard A, et al. Adverse events among medical patients after discharge from hospital. CMAJ 2004;170:345.

31. Kripalani S, Roumie CL, Dalal AK, et al. Effect of a pharmacist intervention on clinically important medication errors after hospital discharge: a randomized trial. Ann Intern Med 2012;157:1.

32. Kripalani S, LeFevre F, Phillips CO, et al. Deficits in communication and information transfer between hospital-based and primary care physicians: implications for patient safety and continuity of care. JAMA 2007;297:831.

33. Roy CL, Poon EG, Karson AS, et al. Patient safety concerns arising from test results that return after hospital discharge. Ann Intern Med 2005;143:121.

34. Walz SE, Smith M, Cox E, et al. Pending laboratory tests and the hospital discharge summary in patients discharged to sub-acute care. J Gen Intern Med 2011;26:393.

35. Were MC, Li X, Kesterson J, et al. Adequacy of hospital discharge summaries in documenting tests with pending results and outpatient follow-up providers. J Gen Intern Med 2009;24:1002.

36. Ong MS, Magrabi F, Jones G, et al. Last orders: follow-up of tests ordered on the day of hospital discharge. Arch Intern Med 2012;172:1347.

37. Moore C, McGinn T, Halm E. Tying up loose ends: discharging patients with unresolved medical issues. Arch Intern Med 2007;167:1305.

38. Hernandez AF, Greiner MA, Fonarow GC, et al. Relationship between early physician follow-up and 30-day readmission among Medicare beneficiaries hospitalized for heart failure. JAMA 2010;303:1716.

39. Misky GJ, Wald HL, Coleman EA. Post-hospitalization transitions: examining the effects of timing of primary care provider follow-up. J Hosp Med 2010;5:392.

40. Sharma G, Kuo YF, Freeman JL, et al. Outpatient follow-up visit and 30-day emergency department visit and readmission in patients hospitalized for chronic obstructive pulmonary disease. Arch Intern Med 2010;170:1664.

41. Doctoroff L, McNally D, Vanka A, et al. Inpatient-outpatient transitions for patients with resident primary care physicians: access and readmission. Am J Med 2014;127:886.e15.

42. Grafft CA, McDonald FS, Ruud KL, et al. Effect of hospital follow-up appointment on clinical event outcomes and mortality. Arch Intern Med 2010;170:955.

43. Field TS, Ogarek J, Garber L, et al. Association of early post-discharge follow-up by a primary care physician and 30-day rehospitalization among older adults. J Gen Intern Med 2015;30:565.

44. Graham KL, Wilker EH, Howell MD, et al. Differences between early and late readmissions among patients: a cohort study. Ann Intern Med 2015;162:741.

45. Forster AJ, Murff HJ, Peterson JF, et al. Adverse drug events occurring following hospital discharge. J Gen Intern Med 2005;20:317.

46. Budnitz DS, Shehab N, Kegler SR, et al. Medication use leading to emergency department visits for adverse drug events in older adults. Ann Intern Med 2007;147:755.

47. Budnitz DS, Pollock DA, Weidenbach KN, et al. National surveillance of emergency department visits for outpatient adverse drug events. JAMA 2006;296:1858.

48. van Walraven C, Forster AJ. Anticoagulation control in the peri-hospitalization period. J Gen Intern Med 2007;22:727.

49. Available at: www.npsf.org/askme3. Accessed April 6, 2009.

50. Campbell SE, Seymour DG, Primrose WR, et al. A systematic literature review of factors affecting outcome in older medical patients admitted to hospital. Age Ageing 2004;33:110.

51. Medicare Hospital Quality Chartbook 2012. Available at: www.cms.gov/Medicare/Quality-Initiatives-Patient-Assessment-Instruments/HospitalQualityInits/Downloads/MedicareHospitalQualityChartbook2012.pdf. Accessed March 25, 2013.

52. Kim CS, Flanders SA. In the clinic. Transitions of care. Ann Intern Med 2013;158:ITC3.

53. Büla CJ, Wietlisbach V, Burnand B, et al. Depressive symptoms as a predictor of 6-month outcomes and services utilization in elderly medical inpatients. Arch Intern Med 2001;161:2609.

54. Strunin L, Stone M, Jack B. Understanding rehospitalization risk: can hospital discharge be modified to reduce recurrent hospitalization? J Hosp Med 2007;2:297.

55. Phillips CO, Wright SM, Kern DE, et al. Comprehensive discharge planning with postdischarge support for older patients with congestive heart failure: a meta-analysis. JAMA 2004;291:1358.

56. Gwadry-Sridhar FH, Flintoft V, Lee DS, et al. A systematic review and meta-analysis of studies comparing readmission rates and mortality rates in patients with heart failure. Arch Intern Med 2004;164:2315.

57. Coleman EA, Wagner EH, Grothaus LC, et al. Predicting hospitalization and functional decline in older health plan enrollees: are administrative data as accurate as self-report? J Am Geriatr Soc 1998;46:419.

58. Mudge AM, Kasper K, Clair A, et al. Recurrent readmissions in medical patients: a prospective study. J Hosp Med 2011;6:61.

59. Billings J, Dixon J, Mijanovich T, et al. Case finding for patients at risk of readmission to hospital: development of algorithm to identify high risk patients. BMJ 2006;333:327.

60. Cornette P, D'Hoore W, Malhomme B, et al. Differential risk factors for early and later hospital readmission of older patients. Aging Clin Exp Res 2005;17:322.

61. Smith DM, Giobbie-Hurder A, Weinberger M, et al. Predicting non-elective hospital readmissions: a multi-site study. Department of Veterans Affairs Cooperative Study Group on Primary Care and Readmissions. J Clin Epidemiol 2000;53:1113.

62. Rodríguez-Artalejo F, Guallar-Castillón P, Herrera MC, et al. Social network as a predictor of hospital readmission and mortality among older patients with heart failure. J Card Fail 2006;12:621.

63. Allaudeen N, Vidyarthi A, Maselli J, et al. Redefining readmission risk factors for general medicine patients. J Hosp Med 2011;6:54.

64. Joynt KE, Orav EJ, Jha AK. Thirty-day readmission rates for Medicare beneficiaries by race and site of care. JAMA 2011;305:675.

65. Baker DW, Gazmararian JA, Williams MV, et al. Functional health literacy and the risk of hospital admission among Medicare managed care enrollees. Am J Public Health 2002;92:1278.

66. Kangovi S, Barg FK, Carter T, et al. Challenges faced by patients with low socioeconomic status during the post-hospital transition. J Gen Intern Med 2014;29:283.

67. Foraker RE, Rose KM, Suchindran CM, et al. Socioeconomic status, Medicaid coverage, clinical

comorbidity, and rehospitalization or death after an incident heart failure hospitalization: Atherosclerosis Risk in Communities cohort (1987 to 2004). Circ Heart Fail 2011;4:308.

68. Kind AJ, Jencks S, Brock J, et al. Neighborhood socioeconomic disadvantage and 30-day rehospitalization: a retrospective cohort study. Ann Intern Med 2014;161:765.

69. Lindquist LA, Baker DW. Understanding preventable hospital readmissions: masqueraders, markers, and true causal factors. J Hosp Med 2011;6:51.

70. Hasan O, Meltzer DO, Shaykevich SA, et al. Hospital readmission in general medicine patients: a prediction model. J Gen Intern Med 2010;25:211.

71. Kansagara D, Englander H, Salanitro A, et al. Risk prediction models for hospital readmission: a systematic review. JAMA 2011;306:1688.

72. Halfon P, Eggli Y, Prêtre-Rohrbach I, et al. Validation of the potentially avoidable hospital readmission rate as a routine indicator of the quality of hospital care. Med Care 2006;44:972.

73. van Walraven C, Bennett C, Jennings A, et al. Proportion of hospital readmissions deemed avoidable: a systematic review. CMAJ 2011;183: E391.

74. van Walraven C, Dhalla IA, Bell C, et al. Derivation and validation of an index to predict early death or unplanned readmission after discharge from hospital to the community. CMAJ 2010;182:551.

75. Donzé JD, Williams MV, Robinson EJ, et al. International Validity of the HOSPITAL Score to Predict 30-Day Potentially Avoidable Hospital Readmissions. JAMA Intern Med 2016;176:496.

76. Southern WN, Nahvi S, Arnsten JH. Increased risk of mortality and readmission among patients discharged against medical advice. Am J Med 2012; 125:594.

77. Hansen LO, Young RS, Hinami K, et al. Interventions to reduce 30-day rehospitalization: a systematic review. Ann Intern Med 2011;155:520.

78. Hesselink G, Schoonhoven L, Barach P, et al. Improving patient handovers from hospital to primary care: a systematic review. Ann Intern Med 2012;157:417.

79. Leppin AL, Gionfriddo MR, Kessler M, et al. Preventing 30-day hospital readmissions: a systematic review and meta-analysis of randomized trials. JAMA Intern Med 2014;174:1095.

80. Mistiaen P, Poot E. Telephone follow-up, initiated by a hospital-based health professional, for postdischarge problems in patients discharged from hospital to home. Cochrane Database Syst Rev 2006;(4):CD004510.

81. Balaban RB, Weissman JS, Samuel PA, et al. Redefining and redesigning hospital discharge to

enhance patient care: a randomized controlled study. J Gen Intern Med 2008;23:1228.

82. Dudas V, Bookwalter T, Kerr KM, et al. The impact of follow-up telephone calls to patients after hospitalization. Am J Med 2001;111:26S.

83. Phatak A, Prusi R, Ward B, et al. Impact of pharmacist involvement in the transitional care of high-risk patients through medication reconciliation, medication education, and postdischarge call-backs (IPITCH Study). J Hosp Med 2016;11:39.

84. Crocker JB, Crocker JT, Greenwald JL. Telephone follow-up as a primary care intervention for postdischarge outcomes improvement: a systematic review. Am J Med 2012;125:915.

85. Stewart S, Pearson S, Horowitz JD. Effects of a home-based intervention among patients with congestive heart failure discharged from acute hospital care. Arch Intern Med 1998;158:1067.

86. Rogers J, Perlic M, Madigan EA. The effect of frontloading visits on patient outcomes. Home Healthc Nurse 2007;25:103.

87. Crossen-Sills J, Toomey I, Doherty M. Strategies to reduce unplanned hospitalizations of home healthcare patients: a STEP-BY-STEP APPROACH. Home Healthc Nurse 2006;24:368.

88. Jerant AF, Azari R, Nesbitt TS. Reducing the cost of frequent hospital admissions for congestive heart failure: a randomized trial of a home telecare intervention. Med Care 2001;39:1234.

89. Chaudhry SI, Phillips CO, Stewart SS, et al. Telemonitoring for patients with chronic heart failure: a systematic review. J Card Fail 2007;13:56.

90. Coleman EA, Parry C, Chalmers S, et al. The care transitions intervention: results of a randomized controlled trial. Arch Intern Med 2006;166:1822.

91. Voss R, Gardner R, Baier R, et al. The care transitions intervention: translating from efficacy to effectiveness. Arch Intern Med 2011;171:1232.

92. Legrain S, Tubach F, Bonnet-Zamponi D, et al. A new multimodal geriatric discharge-planning intervention to prevent emergency visits and rehospitalizations of older adults: the optimization of medication in AGEd multicenter randomized controlled trial. J Am Geriatr Soc 2011;59:2017.

93. Naylor MD, Brooten DA, Campbell RL, et al. Transitional care of older adults hospitalized with heart failure: a randomized, controlled trial. J Am Geriatr Soc 2004;52:675.

94. Stauffer BD, Fullerton C, Fleming N, et al. Effectiveness and cost of a transitional care program for heart failure: a prospective study with concurrent controls. Arch Intern Med 2011;171:1238.

95. Hansen LO, Greenwald JL, Budnitz T, et al. Project BOOST: effectiveness of a multihospital effort to reduce rehospitalization. J Hosp Med 2013;8:421–7.

APPENDIX 1: PROGRAM INITIATIVES

Several program initiatives are underway to investigate and facilitate interventions to promote improved hospital discharge processes. These programs and their Web sites include:

- The National Transitions of Care Coalition— This site offers tools and resources for both patients and providers to help improve the safety of health care transitions. Many of the tools are offered in languages other than English.
- The Institute for Health Care Improvement— This site contains numerous resources about care transitions and other quality-related components of health care in the United States.
- The Care Transitions Program—This site contains information about the Care Transitions Programs and also contains tools for implementing this program. Some features are translated into Spanish and Russian.
- Project BOOST (Society of Hospital Medicine)—This is a step-by-step guide for implementing Project BOOST (Better Outcomes through Optimizing Safe Transitions). Project

BOOST is a mentored implementation program designed to improve transitions from hospital to home. In a pre-post study evaluating this initiative, hospital units that participated in Project BOOST had reduced rates of readmission, with a mean absolute reduction of 2%.[95] Of note, readmission rates in comparison (control) units at the same institutions showed no change in readmission rates. The site also offers extensive information about quality improvement practices.

- Project RED (Re-Engineered Discharge)— This site provides information on the key concepts and primary tools that are the foundation for the National Quality Forum's National Patient Safety Goal on safe discharge. Their toolkit is also available.
- Post-Acute Care Transitions (PACT)Toolkit (Society of Hospital Medicine)— This site offers resources to help optimize transitions between hospitals and skilled nursing facilities.
- The Transitional Care Model—This site contains information about the Transitional Care Model, which uses an advanced practice nurse to deliver and coordinate care across health care settings for geriatric patients.

Index

Note: Page numbers of article titles are in **boldface** type.

A

Accreditation
    and Composite Performance Score, 299
Agreement rates
    and database audit, 295

C

CER. See *Comparative effectiveness research.*
Comparative effectiveness research
    and patient-reported outcomes, 280, 286, 287
Composite measures
    for esophageal cancer resection, 224
    and Society of Thoracic Surgeons, 245–249
    and Society of Thoracic Surgeons General
        Thoracic Surgery Database, 224
Composite Performance Score
    and accreditation, 299
    and European Society of Thoracic Surgeons, 299
CPS. See *Composite Performance Score.*

D

Database audit
    and agreement rates, 295
    and quality metrics, 291–295
    and Society of Thoracic Surgeons General
        Thoracic Surgery Database, 291–295
Database audit in thoracic surgery, **291–296**
Database collaboration
    challenges in, 311
    and European Society of Thoracic Surgeons
        database, 304, 305
    future directions for, 311, 312
    and Society of Thoracic Surgeons General
        Thoracic Surgery Database, 303, 304
    and thoracic surgery, 303–312
    and variable definitions, 306–310

E

Early death
    and avoidance after thoracic surgery, 258, 259
    and causes after thoracic surgery, 258
    conceptual framework for, 258
    and failure-to-rescue, 257–263
    and prevention and rescue, 259
    and rescue after thoracic surgery, 259

Eastern Cooperative Oncology Group
    and outcome measurements, 217
ECOG. See *Eastern Cooperative Oncology Group.*
Endoscopic ultrasound
    and esophageal cancer staging, 236, 237
Enhanced recovery pathway
    and esophageal cancer resection, 223
Esophageal cancer
    and adequate lymphadenectomy, 237–241
    and complete resection, 236–238
    and induction chemoradiation, 240, 241
    and minimally invasive vs. open
        esophagectomy, 274
    and neoadjuvant treatment, 274
    oncologic quality indicators for, 233–241
    and quality of care model, 228
    and stage-based value, 274, 275
    and transhiatal vs. transthoracic
        esophagectomy, 274
    and volume-outcome relationships, 254
Esophageal cancer resection
    and composite measures, 224
    and enhanced recovery pathway, 223
    and operative risk, 222
    and performance measurements, 224
    and postoperative complications, 222, 223
    and preoperative risk, 222
    prolonged hospitalization after, 223
    and risk adjustment, 221–224
Esophageal cancer staging
    and endoscopic ultrasound, 236, 237
    and PET-CT, 236, 237
Esophagectomy
    and failure-to-rescue, 262
    and hospital readmissions, 318
    minimally invasive vs. open, 274
    transhiatal vs. transthoracic, 274
ESOS. See *European Society Objective Score.*
ESTS. See *European Society of Thoracic Surgeons.*
Eurolung
    and European Society of Thoracic Surgeons,
        299–302
Eurolung morbidity scores
    and distribution of complications, 300, 302
European Society Objective Score
    and European Society of Thoracic Surgeons,
        298, 299
European Society of Thoracic Surgeons
    and Composite Performance Score, 299

Moving?

Make sure your subscription moves with you!

To notify us of your new address, find your **Clinics Account Number** (located on your mailing label above your name), and contact customer service at:

Email: journalscustomerservice-usa@elsevier.com

800-654-2452 (subscribers in the U.S. & Canada)
314-447-8871 (subscribers outside of the U.S. & Canada)

Fax number: 314-447-8029

Elsevier Health Sciences Division
Subscription Customer Service
3251 Riverport Lane
Maryland Heights, MO 63043

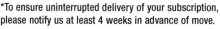

Printed and bound by CPI Group (UK) Ltd, Croydon, CR0 4YY

08/05/2025

01864701-0007